Current Cardiovascular Therapy

Series editor:
Juan Carlos Kaski
Cardiovascular and Cell Sciences Research Institute
St George's University of London
London
UK

Cardiovascular pharmacotherapy is a fast-moving and complex discipline within cardiology in general. New studies, trials and indications are appearing on a regular basis.This series created with the support of the International Society of Cardiovascular Pharmacotherapy (ISCP) is designed to establish the baseline level of knowledge that a cardiovascular professional needs to know on a day-to-day basis. The information within is designed to allow readers to learn quickly and with certainty the mode of action, the possible adverse effects, and the management of patients prescribed these drugs. The emphasis is on current practice, but with an eye to the near-future direction of treatment.This series of titles will be presented as highly practical information, written in a quick-access, no-nonsense format. The emphasis will be on a just-the-facts clinical approach, heavy on tabular material, light on dense prose. The books in the series will provide both an in-depth view of the science and pharmacology behind these drugs and a practical guide to their usage, which is quite unique.Each volume is designed to be between 120 and 250 pages containing practical illustrations and designed to improve understand and practical usage of cardiovascular drugs in specific clinical areas. The books will be priced to attract individuals and presented in a softback format. It will be expected to produce new editions quickly in response to the rapid speed of development of new CV pharmacologic agents.

More information about this series at
http://www.springer.com/series/10472

Hector O. Ventura
Editor

Pharmacologic Trends
of Heart Failure

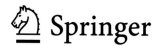

Editor
Hector O. Ventura
Department of Cardiology
Ochsner Health System
New Orleans, LA
USA

Current Cardiovascular Therapy
ISBN 978-3-319-30591-2   ISBN 978-3-319-30593-6   (eBook)
DOI 10.1007/978-3-319-30593-6

Library of Congress Control Number: 2016941739

Printed on acid-free paper

This Springer imprint is published by Springer Nature
The registered company is Springer International Publishing AG Switzerland

Contents

Contributors

Patrick T. Campbell, MD Heart Transplant Institute,
Baptist Health Transplant Institute, Little Rock, AR, USA

Lauren Cooper, MD Division of Cardiology,
Department of Medicine, Duke University Medical Center,
Durham, NC, USA

Clement C. Eiswirth, FACC, FASE Department of Cardiology
Section of Cardiomyopathy and Heart Transplantation,
Ochner Medical Center, New Orleans, LA, USA

Tulane University School of Medicine, New Orleans, LA, USA

Selim R. Krim, MD Department of Cardiology,
John Ochsner Heart and Vascular Institute,
Ochsner Clinic Foundation, New Orleans, LA, USA

Arthur Menezes, MD Department of Cardiology,
John Ochsner Heart and Vascular Institute,
Ochsner Clinic Foundation, New Orleans, LA, USA

Robert J. Mentz, MD Division of Cardiology,
Department of Medicine, Duke University Medical Center,
Durham, NC, USA

Sepehr Saberian, MD Department of Cardiology,
University of Illinois College of Medicine at Peaoria,
Peoria, IL, USA

Hector O. Ventura, MD Division of Cardiology,
John Ochsner Heart and Vascular Institute,
Ochsner Clinic Foundation, New Orleans, LA, USA

Chapter 1
The Established Therapies: HF-PEF and HF-REF

Arthur Menezes, Selim R. Krim, and Hector O. Ventura

Heart Failure with Reduced Ejection Fraction (HFrEF)

Over the last few decades, our understanding of the pathophysiology, and subsequently treatment, of chronic heart failure with reduced ejection fraction (HFrEF) has grown considerably. While diuretics and digoxin were once the pillars of treatment for HFrEF, they did not offer any mortality benefits. The discovery of beta blocker, angiotensin-converting enzyme inhibitors (ACE-I), angiotensin-receptor blockers (ARB's), potassium-sparing diuretics, and their utility in the setting of HFrEF has greatly improved outcomes among these patients.

―――――――

A. Menezes, MD • S.R. Krim, MD
Division of Cardiology, John Ochsner Heart and Vascular Institute, Ochsner Clinic Foundation, 1514 Jefferson Highway, New Orleans, LA 70121, USA

H.O. Ventura, MD (✉)
Division of Cardiology, John Ochsner Heart and Vascular Institute, Ochsner Clinic Foundation, 1514 Jefferson Highway, New Orleans, LA 70121, USA
e-mail: hventura@ochsner.org

H.O. Ventura (ed.), *Pharmacologic Trends of Heart Failure*, Current Cardiovascular Therapy, DOI 10.1007/978-3-319-30593-6_1, © Springer International Publishing Switzerland 2016

Diuretics

Sodium and water retention which result in systemic volume overload are an inevitable sequelae of heart failure and are associated with pulmonary and systemic venous congestion [1]. In the setting of heart failure, alterations in the sympathetic nervous system (SNS), the renin-angiotensin-aldosterone system (RAAS), the vasopressin axis, and vasodilatory/natriuretic pathways lead to sodium and water retention at the level of the renal circulatory system [2].

Loop Diuretics

The use of diuretics among patients with HFrEF who have evidence of fluid overload is recommended to restore and maintain normal volume status [3]. Currently, loop diuretics are the current preferred diuretic agent among most patients with HFrEF. These agents (furosemide, bumetanide, and torsemide) inhibit the reabsorption of sodium, potassium, and chloride in the ascending loop of Henle. The diuretic effects of these drugs depend on its tubular fluid concentration [4, 5]. As a result, higher doses of loop diuretics are required in the setting of severe renal insufficiency or low cardiac output to ensure delivery of sufficient concentrations of the drug to its site of action [6]. The efficacy of loop diuretics also depends on gastrointestinal absorption which can decrease due to bowel wall edema cause by sphlanchnic congestion in the setting of decompensated heart failure. Decreased gastrointestinal absorption and/or insufficient delivery of sufficient drug concentrations to site of action can lead to diuretic resistance. Therefore, appropriate diuretic dosing is vital in maintaining normal volume status among individuals with heart failure.

Resistance to the effects of diuretics can also occur due to post diuretic sodium retention and the braking phenomenon [7]. Since diuretics such as furosemide are short acting, there is a tendency for reabsorption of filtered sodium when there is no longer a diuretic acting in the renal tubule, especially when salt intake is not restricted. Increasing the frequency of diuretic administration reduces the drug-free interval and may be an effective strategy to overcome post-diuretic sodium retention [7]. The braking phenomenon is characterized by a diminished response to loop diuretics over time due to chronic administration. This can be explained in part due to adaptive structural and functional changes in the epithelial cells of the distal convoluted tubules which result in distal reabsorbtion of sodium and decreased sodium excretion [8, 9].

In the setting of diuretic resistance, increasing the dose of the loop diuretic will compensate for the pharmacokinetic and pharmacodynamic changes that occur in CHF and may be an effective strategy [10]. The use of intravenous loop diuretics at a dose higher than the outpatient dose or oral loop diuretics with a higher oral bioavailability than furosemide may be used [11]. Current evidence demonstrates no significant difference in patient symptoms or changes in renal function when loop diuretics were administered as a bolus when compared to continuous infusion, or at a high dose when compared to a low dose [12]. Furthermore, there does not appear to be any difference in the safety and efficacy between bolus injection when compared to continuous infusion of loop diuretics [13].

Thiazide and Thiazide-Type Diuretics

While increasing the dose of the loop diuretic is an effective strategy in overcoming diuretic resistance, there are instances when this approach may not always be successful. The addition of thiazides or thiazide-type diuretics to loop diuretics appear to be highly effective in promoting diuresis among patient resistant to high dose loop diuretics [14]. By decreasing sodium reabsorption in the distal tubules, the addition of thiazides or thiazide-type diuretics potentially antagonize post-diuretic sodium retention and renal adaption to chronic loop diuretic administration [15, 16]. While metolazone is more commonly used in combination with loop diuretics, there is no evidence to support its superiority over other thiazide diuretics [17]. The use of thiazide or thiazide-type diuretics in addition to loop diuretics can significantly increase natriuresis and help maintain a normal volume status [18]. However, there is an increased risk of inducing severe hypokalemia, hyponatremia, hypotension, and worsening renal function [19].

Potassium-Sparing Diuretics

Potassium-sparing diuretics (spironolactone and eplerenone) function by competitively antagonizing the aldosterone receptor. The use of aldosterone receptor antagonists in the setting of HFrEF has been shown to provide a survival benefit [20, 21]. Although only examined in a small number of patients, there is evidence to suggest that the use of ACE-I or ARB's may not uniformly suppress the rennin-angiotensin-aldosterone system. In fact, despite ACE inhibition, elevated levels of plasma aldosterone were observed among 10–38 % of individuals with congestive heart failure [22–24].. This phenomenon is called "aldosterone breakthrough" and may have important clinical consequences especially considering aldosterone's profibrotic action in non-epithelial tissue which may result in cardiac hypertrophy and fibrosis [25]. This would also explain the mortality benefit observed among patients with HFrEF despite treatment with ACE-I or ARB's.

In the Randomized Aldactone Evaluation Study (RALES), the use of spironolactone in patients with HFrEF and NYHA class III to IV demonstrated a 30 % decrease when added to an ACE-I and loop diuretic therapy [26]. Similarly, in the Eplerenone Post-Acute Myocardial Infarction Heart Failure Efficacy and Survival Study (EPHESUS), the use of eplerenone in patients with HFrEF after an acute myocardial infarction (AMI) demonstrated a 15 % decrease in all-cause mortality and a 21 % decrease in sudden cardiac death [27]. Most of the individuals in this study were on an ACE-I or ARB, as well as a beta-blocker. Similar mortality benefits were observed among HfrEF patients using eplerenone in the Eplerenone in Mild Patients Hospitalization and Survival Study in Heart Failure (EMPHASIS-HF) trial in which patients treated eplerenone with HFrEF and mild symptoms (NYHA II) had a reduced risk of death and hospitalization [28]. Similar to RALES and EPHESUS, a majority of the patients in the EMPHASIS-HF trial were concomitantly treated with an ACE-I and/or ARB, and a beta blocker.

It is important to note an increased risk of hyperkalemia among HFrEF patients treated with potassium-sparing diuretics [29]. This risk is increased among individuals with renal dysfunction and there is insufficient data to support the use of potassium-sparing diuretics in patients with a serum creatinine ≥ 2.5 mg/dL (221 μmol/L) or eGFR <30 mL/min per 1.73 m^2 since most of the available trials excluded these patients.

ACE-Inhibitors and ARB's

In patients with HFrEF, maladaptive mechanisms lead to increased RAAS activity, which cause cardiac remodeling and increased sympathetic activation. RAAS activation is sensitive to low cardiac output (CO) and/or low renal perfusion [30]. In early heart failure, a reduced CO prompts RAAS-activated fluid retention, which increases ventricular preload and CO until sufficient CO and renal perfusion is maintained. In the setting of HFrEF, RAAS is persistently activated in an attempt to raise the chronically low CO [31].

Angiotensin I is cleaved by ACE to produce angiotensin II which acts directly on vascular smooth muscle cells to cause vasoconstriction [32]. Angiotensin II also causes vasoconstriction by interacting with the sympathetic nervous system [33]. Angiotensin II also stimulates the production of aldosterone [34] and antidiuretic hormone, [35] which in turn increases volume expansion through sodium and water retention.

ACE-Inhibitors

Unless contraindicated, ACE-I's are recommended in all patients with HFrEF and have been shown to reduce morbidity and mortality. ACE-I's promote sodium excretion by reducing the production of aldosterone and by increasing renal blood flow. This class of drugs also decreases fluid retention by indirectly decreasing circulating levels of antidiuretic hormone. By blocking the effects of ACE and other growth factors on myocytes, ACE-I's are also effective in attenuating cardiac remodeling and left ventricular dysfunction [36, 37]. Finally, by indirectly influencing vascular smooth muscle vasoconstriction and the sympathetic nervous system, ACE-I's reduce preload and afterload, thereby increasing CO in patients with HFrEF [38, 39].

Over the last three decades, there have been multiple studies that have demonstrated a mortality benefit of ACE-I's among patient with HFrEF. The Cooperative North Scandinavian Enalapril Survival Study (CONSENSUS) evaluated the influence of ACE-I (enalapril) on patients with HFrEF with overt CHF symptoms (NYHA class IV) [40]. Among individuals assigned to the treatment arm, there was a significant decrease in mortality compared to the placebo group. Similarly, patients treated with enalapril demonstrated significant improvements in NYHA classification and a reduction in heart size. The Studies of Left Ventricular Dysfunction (SOLVD) trial, unlike the CONSENSUS trial, evaluated the effects of ACE-I (enalapril) on mortality and hospitalization among patients with HFrEF and NYHA functional classes II and III [41]. Treatment with ACE-I instead of placebo resulted in significantly reduced mortality and hospitalization for heart failure among individuals with HFrEF. In fact, even among asymptomatic patients with HFrEF, the use of ACE-I reduced the incidence of heart failure and heart failure related hospitalizations and there was a trend towards fewer cardiovascular deaths among patients receiving enalapril [42].

ARB's

As mentioned earlier, due to the long-term deleterious effects of RAAS in the setting of HFrEF, it remains a viable target for therapy. While ACE-I's have been shown to improve morbidity and mortality, there is evidence to suggest that circulating levels of angiotensin II return to ACE-I pre-treatment levels with long term ACE inhibition. This may be due to non-ACE pathways of angiotensin I metabolism and is known as the "escape phenomenon" [43]. This partly explains the logic behind the development of ARB's. ARB's block the RAAS at the level of the receptors and thereby enable kinin degradation. Moreover, ARB's are theoretically expected to provide the benefits of ACE-I's with fewer of their side effects such as angioedema and cough.

ACE-I's currently remain the first choice for suppression of the RAAS in patients with HFrEF. However, ARB's are an acceptable alternative to reduce morbidity and mortality in patients with HFrEF who are ACE-I intolerant. The Evaluation of Losartan In The Elderly (ELITE) I study was among the first clinical trials to compare an ACE-I (captopril) to an ARB (losartan) in patients with HFrEF [44]. While there was no difference in the primary endpoint, which evaluated increases in serum creatinine between the two groups, the ARB treatment arm had significantly lower rates of all-cause mortality when compared to the ACE-I treatment group. However, it should be noted that the study was not designed to detect a difference in mortality between the two groups. A subsequent trial, the ELITE II study, attempted to compare ACE-I (captopril) to ARB (losartan) with all-cause mortality as the primary end point [45]. The data did not demonstrate any statistically significant difference in all-cause mortality between losartan and captopril among patients with HFrEF with NYHA class II–IV.

While the Valsartan Heart Failure Trial (Val-HeFT) demonstrated that complete blockade of the RAAS by adding valsartan to ACE-I's in patients with HFrEF reduced the combined endpoint of morbidity and mortality, there was no overall mortality benefit. Furthermore, post-hoc analysis demonstrated adverse effects on morbidity and mortality among the subgroup of patients who were already on heart failure drug regimens containing ACE-I's and beta blockers and were started on valsartan [46]. The Candesartan in Heart failure Assessment of Reduction in Mortality and morbidity (CHARM) trial consisted of three simultaneous parallel arms that evaluated the use of ARB (candesartan) versus placebo in different settings of heart failure. The CHARM-Alternative arm of the CHARM trial evaluated efficacy of ARB use in patients with HFrEF who were not receiving ACE-I due to a history of intolerance [47]. There was a statistically significant reduction in cardiovascular death and hospital admission for CHF among patients treated with candesartan compared to those treated with placebo. This suggests that ARB's may be a good alternative to ACE-I's in patients that are ACE-I intolerant. CHARM-Added arm was the only trial to show a reduction in cardiovascular mortality and congestive heart failure hospital admission when candesartan was added to an ACE-I [48]. However, there was no statistically significant difference in deaths from any cause between the groups treated with candesartan when compared to the placebo group. Furthermore, patients treated with dual RAAS therapy had higher rates of withdrawal from the study due to renal dysfunction and hyperkalemia. Due to the lack of evidence demonstrating consistent survival benefits with dual RAAS therapy and an increase in adverse effects, current data does not support concomitant use of ACE-I's and ARB's for the treatment of HFrEF.

Beta-Blockers

The use of beta adrenoceptor blockers in the setting of heart failure was first hypothesized in the 1970s and was widely met with skepticism. However, today, beta blockade is the mainstay therapy in patients with stable HFrEF. Along with the RAAS, the SNS is chronically activated in the setting of heart failure. In the acute setting, these compensatory systems help maintain cardiac output and blood pressure. However, long-term activation of these systems have been shown to have detrimental effects which lead to remodeling of the myocardium and worsening cardiac function [49]. Currently, one of three beta-blockers (bisoprolol, carvedilol, metoprolol succinate) are currently recommended to reduce morbidity and mortality among patients with HFrEF.

The Cardiac Insufficiency Bisoprolol Study II (CIBIS-II) investigated the efficacy of bisoprolol in reducing all-cause mortality among patients with HFrEF who were receiving diuretics and ACE-I's [50]. The trial was stopped prematurely due to a significant decrease in all-cause mortality observed among patients treated with bisoprolol compared to placebo. Similarly, the Metoprolol CR/XL Randomized Intervention Trial in Congestive Heart Failure (MERIT-HF) evaluated the use of metoprolol controlled release/extended release (CR/XL) in addition to standard heart failure therapy in HFrEF patients [51]. Similar to the CIBIS-II trial, the MERIT-HF trial was stopped prematurely due to a significant decrease in all-cause mortality, as well as sudden deaths and deaths from worsening heart failure in the group treated with metoprolol CR/XL when compared to the group treated with placebo. In addition to bisoprolol and metoprolol succinate, when compared to placebo, carvedilol significantly reduced the combined risk of death or hospitalization from HFrEF in the Carvedilol Prospective Randomized Cumulative Survival (COPERNICUS) trial [52].

In the early 1990s, the MDC trial evaluated the effects of metoprolol tartrate on improvements in survival and morbidity among patients with HFeEF secondary to idiopathic dilated cardiomyopathy, when compared to placebo [53]. Patients were initially started at low doses of the beta blocker and doses were gradually up-titrated. Individuals in the treatment arm demonstrated better improvements in ejection fraction, lower pulmonary wedge pressures, and improved exercise times when compared to the placebo group. Despite these results, the Carvedilol Or Metoprolol European Trial (COMET) compared the efficacy of carvedilol versus metoprolol tartrate on all-cause mortality in patients with HFrEF [54]. At the end of the study, patients treated with carvedilol demonstrated significantly lower rates of all-cause mortality when compared to the patients in the metoprolol tartrate arm. This suggests that while metoprolol tartrate and carvedilol share many similar cardiovascular effects, carvedilol is superior to metoprolol tartrate in extending survival in patients with HFrEF. Based on the results from the MERIT-HF trial and the COMET trial, metoprolol succinate, not metoprolol tartrate, is recommended for patients with HFrEF.

Digoxin

Once, digoxin and diuretic therapy were the foundation of heart failure therapy. However, the development of newer, more effective therapies in addition to recent studies evaluating the efficacy of digoxin in the setting of HFrEF have caused it to fall out of favor. Digoxin is a cardiac glycoside that acts by inhibiting the Na-K-ATPase pump in myocardial cells [55]. This results in an increase in intracellular sodium which promotes sodium-calcium exchange and subsequently increased concentrations of intracellular calcium [56]. This increase in intracellular calcium improves myocyte contractility and, as a result, stroke volume and EF.

Digoxin has not been shown to provide any mortality benefit when used in the setting of HFrEF [57]. However, digoxin therapy has been shown to decrease hospitalizations for cardiovascular causes primarily due to a decrease in HF hospitalizations. This is most likely due to it symptomatic benefits in the setting of HF. As a result, current guidelines recommend using digoxin in patients with HFrEF to decrease HF hospitalizations [58].

Results from the Prospective Randomized study Of Ventricular failure and the Efficacy of Digoxin (PROVED) trial suggest that patients withdrawn from digoxin therapy demonstrated worsening maximal exercise capacity when compared to those that were continued on digoxin [59]. Furthermore, in the Randomized Assessment of Digoxin on Inhibitors of Angiotensin-Converting Enzyme

(RADIANCE) study, patients switched from digoxin to placebo experienced worsening heart failure, decreased functional capacity, lower quality-of-life scores, decreased ejection fractions, increases in heart rate, and higher body weights when compared to those individuals continuing to receive digoxin therapy [60]. This suggests that withdrawal of digoxin in patients with HFrEF may result in undesired clinical consequences.

Finally, it should be noted that the narrow therapeutic index of digoxin increase the risk of toxicity and adverse effects. Digoxin is mainly excreted by the kidneys and as a result, impaired renal function can lead to higher plasma concentrations [61]. Congestive heart failure and advanced age can also reduce the volume of distribution of the drug and increase the risk of toxicity. Other causes that can precipitate digoxin toxicity include hypokalemia, hypomagnesemia, hypocalcemia, medication interaction, as well as hypothyroidism [62, 63].

Hydralazine and Isosorbide Dinitrate

The simultaneous use of hydralazine and isosorbide dinitrate (H-ISDN) in patients with HFrEF was first studied in 1977 [64]. The findings demonstrated a 36 % decrease in left ventricular filling pressures, a 58 % increase in cardiac index, and a 34 % decrease in systemic vascular resistance. These findings lead to the formal evaluation of the effect of H-ISDN on mortality in patients with HFrEF.

The first Vasodilator-Heart Failure Trial (V-HeFT I) compared H-ISDN or prazosin to placebo in over 600 men with HFrEF [65]. H-ISDN was associated with a trend towards decreased mortality when compared to placebo. Additionally, H-ISDN was associated with improvement in left ventricular ejection at 8 weeks and 1 year. The V-HeFT II trial compared H-ISDN and enalapril among patient with HFrEF [66]. After 2 years, there was significantly lower mortality in the enalapril arm. However, when compared to enalapril, treatment with H-ISDN was associated with greater improvements in body oxygen consumption at peak exercise and left ventricular ejection fraction.

The African-American heart failure trial compared treatment with H-ISDN to placebo among black patients with HFrEF and NYHA III or IV symptoms. The study was terminated early due to significantly higher mortality rates in the placebo group compared to the group treated with H-ISDN. As a result, among African-American patients with HFrEF and NYHA III or IV symptoms receiving optimal therapy with ACE-I and beta-blockers (unless contraindicated), H-ISDN is now recommended to reduce morbidity and mortality [67, 68].

Conclusions

Current heart failure therapy is mainly targeted towards HFrEF. While digoxin and diuretics were once the mainstay therapy for HFrEF, newer classes of drugs have emerged that have proven to confer mortality and morbidity benefits. Advances in science and research impart promises of even better future therapies for the management of HFrEF.

Heart Failure with Preserved Ejection Fraction (HFpEF)

HF with preserved ejection fraction (HFpEF) represents nearly half of the five million cases of HF in the United States [69–71] and with the aging of the population its prevalence will likely continue to rise. Unlike patients with HFrEF where advances in therapy have led to significant improvement of outcomes, owing to a lack of randomized trials patient with HFpEF remain at a high risk with an estimated five mortality of 65 % [70, 71]. Although not fully understood, current available literature suggests that mortality in HFpEF patients seem to be driven by the coexisting comorbidities. In this regard, the Acute Decompensated Heart Failure National Registry (ADHERE) study showed that 91 % of patients with HFpEF had a diagnosis of hypertension, CAD, or diabetes [72]. In addition, HFpEF patients are more likely to be older, females and have atrial fibrillation when compared to HFrEF patients [58, 73]. Most of the data for treating HFpEF is derived from smaller studies and expert opinion. This section will summarize available data focusing on HFpEF therapy and recommended approach and rationale for the management of HFpEF.

Diuretics

Similar to HFrEF, diuretics are commonly used to relieve congestion with no mortality benefit. The Hong Kong Diastolic HF study is the only randomized trial to date that assessed the efficacy of diuretics in HFpEF patients [74]. Although no mortality benefit was shown, after 52 weeks of therapy in 150 patients with HFpEF, diuretics significantly improved symptoms, quality of life as assessed by 6-min walk test. Interestingly no benefit was shown with the addition of an angiotensin converting enzyme (Ramipril) or angiotensin receptor blocker (Irbesartan). Another study showed that chlorthalidone was associated with a reduction in the incidence of new-onset hospitalization in patients with HFPEF significantly compared to patients treated with calcium channel blockers or alpha receptor blockers [75]. The same study also suggested that diuretics are associated with a reduction in the incidence of new onset HFpEF when compared to ACE's. (ALLHAT).

In this regard, recent ACC/AHA HF guidelines give a 1C recommendation for diuretic use in patients with HFPEF [58].

ACEI's and ARB's

Although inhibition of the RAAS system has shown to be beneficial in the treatment of HFpEF associated comorbid condition such as hypertension, diabetes and coronary artery disease, ACEI's and ARB therapy have failed to show any mortality benefit in HFpEF. In the Candesartan in Heart failure: Assessment of Reduction in Mortality and morbidity (CHARM-Preserved), a multicenter, double-blind, international trial, candesartan was compared to placebo in 3023 patients with HF-pEF (EF, ≥ 40 %; mean EF, 54 %) [76]. After a mean follow-up duration of 36 months, no significant difference was found in composite outcome of cardiovascular death or admission to hospital for HF between the two groups (22 % in the candesartan group, 24 % in the placebo group; HR, 0.89; 95 % CI, 0.77–1.03; $P=0.118$). Likewise, the Perindopril in Elderly People with Chronic Heart Failure study randomized 850 HFpEF patients to either Perindopril or placebo [77]. After a mean follow-up of 26 months, no difference in all-cause mortality or unplanned HF-related hospitalization was found between the two groups. Finally, the Irbesartan in Heart Failure with Preserved Ejection Fraction Study (I-PRESERVE) randomized 4128 HFpEF patients to either Irbesartan or placebo with a mean follow up duration of 49 months [78]. Again no difference in the primary outcome was seen between the two groups (composite of death from any cause or hospitalization for cardiovascular causes). Additionally, there were no differences in improvement of quality of life at 6 months as assessed by the Minnesota Living with Heart Failure scale between the two groups.

Beta Blockers

Beta blockers play an essential role in controlling tachycardia, reducing myocardial oxygen demand, and regression of LVH [79, 80]. In this regard, in the Swedish Doppler

Echocardiographic study, 113 symptomatic HF patients with preserved left ventricular ejection fraction, and abnormal diastolic function were randomized in a double blind fashion to carvedilol or placebo with echocardiographic assessment at baseline and 6 months [81]. Carvedilol resulted in a significant improvement in the E/A ratio, but no significant improvement in other echocardiographic parameters of diastolic function such as deceleration time, isovolumic relaxation time, or pulmonary vein flow velocity. Two other important studies evaluating the clinical efficacy of beta blockers in HFpEF showed mixed results. First, in the Study of the Effects of Nebivolol Intervention on Outcomes and Rehospitalisation in Seniors with Heart Failure (SENIORS), 2128 patients ≥70 years of age with history of HF (with both HFpEF and HFrEF) were randomly assigned Nebivolol or placebo [82]. After a mean follow-up of 21 months, a statistically significant reduction in the primary outcome of all cause mortality or cardiovascular hospital admission (31 % vs. 35 %; HR, 0.86; 95 % CI, 0.74–0.99; $P = .039$) was shown in the Nebivolol group when compared to placebo. Although a minority of patients included in this study had preserved LV function, the effect of nebivolol on the primary outcome was comparable in patients with preserved and impaired LVEF [83].

Conversely, in the Organized Program to Initiate Lifesaving Treatment in Hospitalized Patients with Heart Failure registry (OPTIMIZE-HF), 7,154 patients hospitalized with heart failure and eligible for beta-blockers, Beta blockers were associated with reduced mortality (adjusted hazard ratios of 0.77; 95 % CI: 0.68–0.87) for mortality and rehospitalization rates (HR of 0.89 (95 % CI: 0.80–0.99) in patients with HFrEF but no improvement in either mortality (HR of 0.94; 95 % CI: 0.84–1.07) or rehospitalization (HR of 0.98; 95 % CI: 0.90–1.06) were shown in HFpEF patients [84]. These results were corroborated by the recently published Japanese Diastolic Heart Failure (J-DHF) study where 245 patients with HF and LVEF

>40 % were randomly assigned to either carvedilol or placebo [85]. After a median follow-up of 3.2 years, no significant differences in the primary endpoint (composite of cardiovascular death and hospitalization for HF) between the carvedilol and the control group.

In summary, beta blockers are commonly used in the treatment of atrial fibrillation, coronary artery disease and HTN all contributing factors for HFpEF and given the limited data on their efficacy in HFpEF, the current ACC/AHA guidelines give a IIa recommendation (level of evidence C) recommendation for their use in patient with HTN and HFpEF [58].

Calcium Channel Blockers (CCB)

The role of CCB in HFPEF has been very limited with no large randomized clinical trials available. Moreover, most published studies have focused on special populations such as patients with hypertrophic cardiomyopathy (HCM) [86]. Nevertheless, most of the evidence suggests that in addition to slowing the heart rate, CCB enhance left ventricular relaxation "lusitropic effect" and diastolic filling. In this regard, in a study of 55 patients with HCM, treatment with verapamil (360–480 mg/day) for 1–4 weeks was associated an increase in peak LV diastolic filling rate and symptomatic improvement on graded exercise testing [87]. Similarly, a small randomized study of 20 patients with HFpEF, verapamil was associated with significant improvement of symptoms of HF and increased LV diastolic filling rate and treadmill exercise time when compared to placebo [88].

Aldosterone Antagonists

Evidence from animal studies suggests that aldosterone antagonists improve left ventricular diastolic dysfunction by reducing left ventricular mass and fibrosis both major factors contributing to myocardial stiffness and diastolic dysfunction [89]. In a small randomized, double-blind, placebo-controlled trial of 44 patients with HFpEF, although a significant reduction in serum markers of collagen turnover and improvement in echocardiographic measures of diastolic function was shown with eplerenone no significant improvement in exercise capacity was observed when compared to placebo [90].

Similarly, in the Aldo-DHF trial, a study that assessed the efficacy of spironolactone in 422 patients with HFpEF, no effects on maximal exercise capacity improvement, symptoms relief, or quality of life were seen [91]. The Treatment of Preserved Cardiac Function Heart Failure with an Aldosterone Antagonist (TOPCAT) trial is the largest study to date assessing the clinical efficacy of spironolactone in an exclusive cohort of HFpEF patients [92]. Hospitalization for HF was less common in the spironolactone group when compared to the placebo group (12 % vs. 14.2%; hazard ratio 0.83; 95 % CI, 0.69–0.99). Second, higher rates of hyperkalemia (18.7 versus 9.1%) and increased creatinine were observed in the spironolactone group compared to the placebo group. Third, among patients in whom the diagnosis of HF was confirmed by elevated BNP or NT-proBNP levels, spironolactone was associated with a reduction in the primary outcome.

In summary, in contrast to HFREF where clear improved survival has been shown, therapy aiming at neuro-hormonal blockade failed to show mortality benefit in HFPEF patients. Current ACC/AHA guidelines recommend treating associated comorbidities such as hypertension, CAD, diabetes, and chronic kidney disease using current available evidence based medicine (Tables 1.1 and 1.2).

TABLE 1.1 ACC/AHA recommendations for pharmacology therapy for HFrEF

Therapy	Indications/use	Recommendation/ level of evidence
Diuretics	Diuretics are recommended in patients with HFrEF with fluid retention IC	Class I/LOE C
Beta blockers	Use of 1 of the 3 beta blockers proven to reduce mortality is recommended for all stable patients IA	Class I/LOE A
ACEI's	ACE inhibitors are recommended for all patients with HFrEF IA	Class I/LOE A
ARBs	ARBs are recommended in patients with HFrEF who are ACE inhibitor intolerant	Class I/LOE A
	ARBs are reasonable as alternatives to ACE inhibitor as first line therapy in HFrEF	Class IIa/LOE A
	The addition of an ARB may be considered in persistently symptomatic patients with HFrEF on GDMT	Class IIb/LOE A
Aldosterone antagonists	Use in patients with NYHA class II-IV HF who have LVEF ≤35 %	Class I/LOE A
	Use in patients following an acute MI who have LVEF ≤40 % with symptoms of HF or Diabetes mellitus	Class I/LOE B
Hydralazine and Isosorbide Dinitrate	The combination of hydralazine and isosorbide dinitrate is recommended for African-Americans, with NYHA class III–IV HFrEF on GDMT	Class I/LOE A
	A combination of hydralazine and isosorbide dinitrate may be beneficial in patients with HFrEF who cannot be given ACE inhibitors or ARBs	Class IIa/LOE B
Digoxin	Digoxin can be beneficial in patients with HFrEF	Class IIa/LOE B

Adapted from 2013 ACCF/AHA Guideline for the Management of Heart Failure [58]

Table 1.2 ACC/AHA recommendations for pharmacology therapy for HFpEF

Therapy	Indication/use	Recommendation/level of evidence
Diuretics	Use for relief of symptoms due to volume overload IC	Class I, LOE C
Beta blockers	Use for hypertension in HFpEF IIa C	Class IIa, LOE C
ARBs	May be used for hypertension in HFpEF Can be considered to decrease hospitalizations in HFpEF patients	Class IIa/LOE C Class IIb/LOE B
ACEI's	Can be used for hypertension in HFpEF	Class IIa/LOE C

Adapted from 2013 ACCF/AHA Guideline for the Management of Heart Failure [58]

References

1. Shchekochikhin D, Al Ammary F, Lindenfeld JA. Role of diuretics and ultrafiltration in congestive heart failure. Pharmaceuticals (Basel). 2013;6(7):851–66.
2. Schrier RW, Abraham WT. Hormones and hemodynamics in heart failure. N Engl J Med. 1999;341:577–85.
3. Cody RJ, Kubo SH, Pickworth KK. Diuretic treatment for the sodium retention of congestive heart failure. Arch Intern Med. 1994;154(17):1905–14.
4. Odlind B, Beermann B. Renal tubular secretion and effects of furosemide. Clin Pharmacol Ther. 1980;27(6):784–90.
5. Odlind B, Beermann B, Lindström B. Coupling between renal tubular secretion and effect of bumetanide. Clin Pharmacol Ther. 1983;34(6):805–9.
6. Risler T, Schwab A, Kramer B, et al. Comparative pharmacokinetics and pharmacodynamics of loop diuretics in renal failure. Cardiology. 1994;84 Suppl 2:155–61.
7. Ellison DH. Diuretic resistance: physiology and therapeutics. Semin Nephrol. 1999;19(6):581–97.

8. Kaissling B, Bachmann S, Kriz W. Structural adaptation of the distal convoluted tubule to prolonged furosemide treatment. Am J Physiol. 1985;248:F374–81.

9. Felker GM, O'Connor CM, Braunwald E, et al. Loop diuretics in acute decompensated heart failure: necessary? Evil? A necessary evil? Circ Heart Fail. 2009;2(1):56–62.

10. De Bruyne LK. Mechanisms and management of diuretic resistance in congestive heart failure. Postgrad Med J. 2003;79:268–71.

11. Brater DC, Day B, Burdette A, et al. Bumetanide and furosemide in heart failure. Kidney Int. 1984;26(2):183–9.

12. Felker GM, Lee KL, Bull DA, et al. Diuretic strategies in patients with acute decompensated heart failure. N Engl J Med. 2011;364:797–805.

13. Wu MY, Chang NC, Su CL, et al. Loop diuretic strategies in patients with acute decompensated heart failure: a meta-analysis of randomized controlled trials. J Crit Care. 2014;29(1):2–9.

14. Jentzer JC, DeWald TA, Hernandez AF. Combination of loop diuretics with thiazide-type diuretics in heart failure. J Am Coll Cardiol. 2010;56(19):1527–34.

15. Ellison DH. The physiologic basis of diuretic synergism: its role in treating diuretic resistance. Cardiology. 2001;96:132–43.

16. Dormans TP, Gerlag PG. Combination of high-dose furosemide and hydrochlorothiazide in the treatment of refractory congestive heart failure. Eur Heart J. 1996;17:1867–74.

17. Channer KS, McLean KA, Lawson-Matthews P, et al. Combination diuretic treatment in severe heart failure: a randomised controlled trial. Br Heart J. 1994;71:146–50.

18. Mouallem M, Brif I, Mayan H, Farfel Z. Prolonged therapy by the combination of furosemide and thiazides in refractory heart failure and other fluid retaining conditions. Int J Cardiol. 1995; 50:89–94.

19. Rosenberg J, Gustafsson F, Galatius S, et al. Combination therapy with metolazone and loop diuretics in outpatients with refractory heart failure: an observational study and review of the literature. Cardiovasc Drugs Ther. 2005;19(4):301–6.

20. Pitt B, Zannad F, Remme WJ, et al. The effect of spironolactone on morbidity and mortality in patients with severe heart failure: Randomized Aldactone Evaluation Study Investigators. N Engl J Med. 1999;341:709–17.

21. Ezekowitz JA, McAlister FA. Aldosterone blockade and left ventricular dysfunction: a systematic review of randomized clinical trials. Eur Heart J. 2009;30:469–77.

22. MacFadyen RJ, Lee AF, Morton JJ, et al. How often are angiotensin II and aldosterone concentrations raised during chronic ACE inhibitor treatment in cardiac failure? Heart. 1999;82: 57–61.
23. Lee AF, MacFadyen RJ, Struthers AD. Neurohormonal reactivation in heart failure patients on chronic ACE inhibitor therapy: a longitudinal study. Eur J Heart Fail. 1999;1:401–6.
24. Cicoira M, Zanolla L, Franceschini L, et al. Relation of aldosterone "escape" despite angiotensin-converting enzyme inhibitor administration to impaired exercise capacity in chronic congestive heart failure secondary to ischemic or idiopathic dilated cardiomyopathy. Am J Cardiol. 2002;89:403–7.
25. Bomback AS, Klemmer PJ. The incidence and implications of aldosterone breakthrough. Nat Clin Pract Nephrol. 2007;3(9): 486–92.
26. Pitt B, Zannad F, Remme WJ, et al. The effect of spironolactone on morbidity and mortality in patients with severe heart failure. Randomized Aldactone Evaluation Study Investigators. N Engl J Med. 1999;341:709.
27. Pitt B, Remme W, Zannad F, et al. Eplerenone, a selective aldosterone blocker, in patients with left ventricular dysfunction after myocardial infarction. N Engl J Med. 2003;348:1309–21.
28. Zannad F, McMurray JJ, Krum H, et al. Eplerenone in patients with systolic heart failure and mild symptoms. N Engl J Med. 2011;364:11.
29. Lee KK, Shilane D, Hlatky MA, et al. Effectiveness and safety of spironolactone for systolic heart failure. Am J Cardiol. 2013; 112(9):1427–32.
30. Andrew P. Renin-angiotensin-aldosterone activation in heart failure, aldosterone escape. Chest. 2002;122(2):755.
31. Weber KT. Aldosterone in congestive heart failure. N Engl J Med. 2001;345:1689–97.
32. Kanaide H, Ichiki T, Nishimura J, et al. Cellular mechanism of vasoconstriction induced by angiotensin II: it remains to be determined. Circ Res. 2003;93(11):1015–7.
33. Phillips MI, Sumners C. Angiotensin II in central nervous system physiology. Regul Pept. 1998;78(1–3):1–11.
34. Hattangady NG, Olala LO, Bollag WB, et al. Acute and chronic regulation of aldosterone production. Mol Cell Endocrinol. 2012;350(2):151–62.
35. Qadri F, Culman J, Veltmar A, et al. Angiotensin II-induced vasopressin release is mediated through alpha-1 adrenoceptors

and angiotensin II AT1 receptors in the supraoptic nucleus. J Pharmacol Exp Ther. 1993;267(2):567–74.

36. Brower GL, Levick SP, Janicki JS. Inhibition of matrix metallo-proteinase activity by ACE inhibitors prevents left ventricular remodeling in a rat model of heart failure. Am J Physiol Heart Circ Physiol. 2007;292(6):H3057–64.

37. Greenberg BH. Effects of angiotensin converting enzyme inhibitors on remodeling in clinical trials. J Card Fail. 2002;8(6 Suppl):S486–90.

38. Gavras H, Faxon DP, Berkoben J, et al. Angiotensin converting enzyme inhibition in patients with congestive heart failure. Circulation. 1978;58:770–6.

39. Pepi M, Tamborini G, Maltagliati A, et al. Effects of acute angiotensin-converting enzyme inhibition on diastolic ventricular interaction in the dilated heart. Clin Cardiol. 2003; 26(9):424–30.

40. CONSENSUS Trial Study Group. Effects of enalapril on mortality in severe congestive heart failure: results of the Cooperative North Scandinavian Enalapril Survival Study (CONSENSUS). N Engl J Med. 1987;316:1429–35.

41. The SOLVD Investigators. Effect of enalapril on survival in patients with reduced left ventricular ejection fractions and congestive heart failure. N Engl J Med. 1991;325:293–302.

42. The SOLVD Investigators. Effect of enalapril on mortality and the development of heart failure in asymptomatic patients with reduced left ventricular ejection fractions. N Engl J Med. 1992;327:685–91.

43. Givertz MM. Manipulation of the renin-angiotensin system. Circulation. 2001;104(5):E14–8.

44. Pitt B, Segal R, Martinez FA, et al. Randomised trial of losartan versus captopril in patients over 65 with heart failure (Evaluation of Losartan in the Elderly Study, ELITE). Lancet. 1997;349(9054): 747–52.

45. Pitt B, Poole-Wilson PA, Segal R, et al. Effect of losartan compared with captopril on mortality in patients with symptomatic heart failure: randomised trial – the Losartan Heart Failure Survival Study ELITE II. Lancet. 2000;355(9215):1582–7.

46. Cohn JN, Tognoni G. A randomized trial of the angiotensin-receptor blocker valsartan in chronic heart failure. N Engl J Med. 2001;345(23):1667–75.

47. Granger CB, McMurray JJ, Yusuf S, et al. Effects of candesartan in patients with chronic heart failure and reduced left-ventricular

systolic function intolerant to angiotensin-converting-enzyme inhibitors: the CHARM-Alternative trial. Lancet. 2003;362(9386): 772–6.

48. Mcmurray JJ, Ostergren J, Swedberg K, et al. Effects of candes-artan in patients with chronic heart failure and reduced leftven-tricular systolic function taking angiotensin converting enzyme inhibitors: the CHARM-Added trial. Lancet. 2003;362:767–71.

49. Squire IB, Barnett DB. The rational use of beta-adrenoceptor blockers in the treatment of heart failure. The changing face of an old therapy. Br J Clin Pharmacol. 2000;49(1):1–9.

50. The Cardiac Insufficiency Bisoprolol Study II (CIBIS-II): a ran-domised trial. Lancet. 1999;353:9–13.

51. Effect of metoprolol CR/XL in chronic heart failure: Metoprolol CR/XL Randomised Intervention Trial in Congestive Heart Failure (MERIT-HF). Lancet. 1999;353:2001–7.

52. Packer M, Fowler MB, Roecker EB, et al. Effect of carvedilol on the morbidity of patients with severe chronic heart failure: results of the carvedilol prospective randomized cumulative survival (COPERNICUS) study. Circulation. 2002;106(17): 2194–9.

53. Waagstein F, Bristow MR, Swedberg K, et al. Beneficial effects of metoprolol in idiopathic dilated cardiomyopathy. Metoprolol in Dilated Cardiomyopathy (MDC) Trial Study Group. Lancet. 1993;342(8885):1441–6.

54. Poole-Wilson PA, Swedberg K, Cleland JG, et al. Comparison of carvedilol and metoprolol on clinical outcomes in patients with chronic heart failure in the Carvedilol Or Metoprolol European Trial (COMET): randomised controlled trial. Lancet. 2003;362(9377):7–13.

55. Smith TW. Digitalis. Mechanisms of action and clinical use. N Engl J Med. 1988;318:358.

56. McMahon WS, Holzgrefe HH, Walker JD, et al. Cellular basis for improved left ventricular pump function after digoxin therapy in experimental left ventricular failure. J Am Coll Cardiol. 1996;28:495.

57. The Digitalis Investigation Group. The effect of digoxin on mor-tality and morbidity in patients with heart failure. N Engl J Med. 1997;336:525–33.

58. Yancy CW, Jessup M, Bozkurt B, Butler J, Casey Jr DE, Drazner MH, Fonarow GC, Geraci SA, Horwich T, Januzzi JL, Johnson MR, Kasper EK, Levy WC, Masoudi FA, McBride PE, McMurray JJ, Mitchell JE, Peterson PN, Riegel B, Sam F, Stevenson LW,

Tang WH, Tsai EJ, Wilkoff BL. 2013 ACCF/AHA Guideline for the Management of Heart Failure. A Report of the American College of Cardiology Foundation/American Heart Association Task Force on Practice Guidelines. J Am Coll Cardiol. 2013; 62(16):e147–239.

59. Uretsky BF, Young JB, Shahidi FE, et al. Randomized study assessing the effect of digoxin withdrawal in patients with mild to moderate chronic congestive heart failure: results of the PROVED trial. PROVED Investigative Group. J Am Coll Cardiol. 1993;22(4):955–62.

60. Packer M, Gheorghiade M, Young JB, et al. Withdrawal of digoxin from patients with chronic heart failure treated with angiotensin-converting-enzyme inhibitors. RADIANCE Study. N Engl J Med. 1993;329(1):1–7.

61. Yang EH, Shah S, Criley JM. Digitalis toxicity: a fading but crucial complication to recognize. Am J Med. 2012;125(4):337–43.

62. Lip GY, Metcalfe MJ, Dunn FG. Diagnosis and treatment of digoxin toxicity. Postgrad Med J. 1993;69(811):337–9.

63. Currie GM, Wheat JM, Kiat H. Pharmacokinetic considerations for digoxin in older people. Open Cardiovasc Med J. 2011;5:130–5.

64. Massie B, Chatterjee K, Werner J, et al. Hemodynamic advantage of combined administration of hydralazine orally and nitrates nonparenterally in the vasodilator therapy of chronic heart failure. Am J Cardiol. 1977;40:794–801.

65. Cohn JN, Archibald DG, Ziesche S, et al. Effect of vasodilator therapy on mortality in chronic congestive heart failure: results of a Veterans Administration cooperative study. N Engl J Med. 1986;314:1547–52.

66. Cohn JN, Johnson G, Ziesche S, et al. A comparison of enalapril with hydralazine-isosorbide dinitrate in the treatment of chronic congestive heart failure. N Engl J Med. 1991;325(5):303–10.

67. Taylor AL, Ziesche S, Yancy C, et al. Combination of isosorbide dinitrate and hydralazine in blacks with heart failure. N Engl J Med. 2004;351:2049–57.

68. Carson P, Ziesche S, Johnson G, et al. Vasodilator-Heart Failure Trial Study Group. Racial differences in response to therapy for heart failure: analysis of the vasodilator-heart failure trials. J Card Fail. 1999;5:178–87.

69. Owan TE, Hodge DO, Herges RM, Jacobsen SJ, Roger VL, Redfield MM. Trends in prevalence and outcome of heart failure with preserved ejection fraction. N Engl J Med. 2006; 355(3):251–9.

70. Redfield MM, Jacobsen SJ, Burnett Jr JC, Mahoney DW, Bailey KR, Rodeheffer RJ. Burden of systolic and diastolic ventricular dysfunction in the community: appreciating the scope of the heart failure epidemic. JAMA. 2003;289(2):194–202.
71. Zile MR, Brutsaert DL. New concepts in diastolic dysfunction and diastolic heart failure; part I: diagnosis, prognosis, and measurements of diastolic function. Circulation. 2002;105:1387–93.
72. Yancy CW, Lopatin M, Stevenson LW, De Marco T, Fonarow GC. Clinical presentation, management, and in-hospital outcomes of patients admitted with acute decompensated heart failure with preserved systolic function: a report from the Acute Decompensated Heart Failure National Registry (ADHERE) Database. J Am Coll Cardiol. 2006;47(1):76–84.
73. Lam CS, Donal E, Kraigher-Krainer E, Vasan RS. Epidemiology and clinical course of heart failure with preserved ejection fraction. Eur J Heart Fail. 2011;13(1):18–28.
74. Yip GW, Wang M, Wang T, et al. The Hong Kong diastolic heart failure study: a randomised controlled trial of diuretics, irbesartan and ramipril on quality of life, exercise capacity, left ventricular global and regional function in heart failure with a normal ejection fraction. Heart. 2008;94(5):573–80.
75. Davis BR, Kostis JB, Simpson LM, et al. Heart failure with preserved and reduced left ventricular ejection fraction in the antihypertensive and lipid-lowering treatment to prevent heart attack trial. Circulation. 2008;118(22):2259–67.
76. Yusuf S, Pfeffer MA, Swedberg K, et al; CHARM Investigators and Committees. Effects of candesartan in patients with chronic heart failure and preserved left-ventricular ejection fraction: the CHARM-Preserved Trial. Lancet. 2003;362(9386):777–81.
77. Cleland JG, Tendera M, Adamus J, Freemantle N, Polonski L, Taylor J; PEP-CHF Investigators. The perindopril in elderly people with chronic heart failure (PEP-CHF) study. Eur Heart J. 2006;27(19):2338–45.
78. Massie BM, Carson PE, McMurray JJ, et al; I-PRESERVE Investigators. Irbesartan in patients with heart failure and preserved ejection fraction. N Engl J Med. 2008;359(23):2456–67.
79. Bonow RO, Udelson JE. Left ventricular diastolic dysfunction as a cause of congestive heart failure. Mechanisms and management. Ann Intern Med. 1992;117(6):502.
80. Brutsaert DL, Sys SU, Gillebert TC. Diastolic failure: pathophysiology and therapeutic implications. J Am Coll Cardiol. 1993;22(1):318.

81. Bergström A, Andersson B, Edner M, Nylander E, Persson H, Dahlström U. Effect of carvedilol on diastolic function in patients with diastolic heart failure and preserved systolic function. Results of the Swedish Doppler-echocardiographic study (SWEDIC). Eur J Heart Fail. 2004;6(4):453.

82. Flather MD, Shibata MC, Coats AJ, et al. Randomized trial to determine the effect of nebivolol on mortality and cardiovascular hospital admission in elderly patients with heart failure (SENIORS). Eur Heart J. 2005;26:215.

83. van Veldhuisen DJ, Cohen-Solal A, Böhm M, et al. Beta-blockade with nebivolol in elderly heart failure patients with impaired and preserved left ventricular ejection fraction: data from SENIORS (Study of Effects of Nebivolol Intervention on Outcomes and Rehospitalization in Seniors With Heart Failure). J Am Coll Cardiol. 2009;53:2150.

84. Hernandez AF, Hammill BG, O'Connor CM, et al. Clinical effectiveness of beta-blockers in heart failure: findings from the OPTIMIZE-HF (Organized Program to Initiate Lifesaving Treatment in Hospitalized Patients with Heart Failure) Registry. J Am Coll Cardiol. 2009;53:184.

85. Yamamoto K, Origasa H, Hori M, J-DHF Investigators. Effects of carvedilol on heart failure with preserved ejection fraction: the Japanese Diastolic Heart Failure Study (J-DHF). Eur J Heart Fail. 2013;15(1):110–8.

86. Hopf R, Kaltenbach M. 10-year results and survival of patients with hypertrophic cardiomyopathy treated with calcium antagonists. Z Kardiol. 1987;76 Suppl 3:137.

87. Bonow RO, Dilsizian V, Rosing DR, Maron BJ, Bacharach SL, Green MV. Verapamil-induced improvement in left ventricular diastolic filling and increased exercise tolerance in patients with hypertrophic cardiomyopathy: short- and long-term effects. Circulation. 1985;72(4):853.

88. Setaro JF, Zaret BL, Schulman DS, Black HR, Soufer R. Usefulness of verapamil for congestive heart failure associated with abnormal left ventricular diastolic filling and normal left ventricular systolic performance. Am J Cardiol. 1990; 66(12):981.

89. Lacolley P, Safar ME, Lucet B, Ledudal K, Labat C, Benetos A. Prevention of aortic and cardiac fibrosis by spironolactone in old normotensive rats. J Am Coll Cardiol. 2001;37:662e7.

90. Deswal A, Richardson P, Bozkurt B, Mann DL. Results of the Randomized Aldosterone Antagonism in heart failure with Preserved Ejection Fraction trial (RAAM-PEF). J Card Fail. 2011;17(8):634–42.

91. Edelmann F, Wachter R, Schmidt AG, et al. Effect of spironolactone on diastolic function and exercise capacity in patients with heart failure with preserved ejection fraction: the Aldo-DHF randomized controlled trial. J Am Med Assoc. 2013;309(8): 781–91.

92. Pitt B, Pfeffer MA, Assmann SF, Boineau R, Anand IS, Claggett B, Clausell N, Desai AS, Diaz R, Fleg JL, Gordeev I, Harty B, Heitner JF, Kenwood CT, Lewis EF, O'Meara E, Probstfield JL, Shaburishvili T, Shah SJ, Solomon SD, Sweitzer NK, Yang S, McKinlay SM, TOPCAT Investigators. Spironolactone for heart failure with preserved ejection fraction. N Engl J Med. 2014;370(15):1383.

Chapter 2
Novel Therapies for the Prevention and Management of Acute Decompensated Heart Failure

Patrick T. Campbell and Sepehr Saberian

Acute decompensated heart failure continues to be a leading cause of hospital admissions in the U.S. and is the leading cause of hospitalization in patients >65 years of age [1]. Over the past three decades significant advances in understanding the complex pathophysiology has lead to the development of medical therapies that have improved outcome, unfortunately the overall mortality rate remains staggeringly high, 50 % at 5 years [2]. Hospitalizations for acute decompensated heart failure (ADHF) are a huge burden to the already over taxed health care system. Even with the advances in the medical therapies, the 30-day readmission rate for ADHF is 25 % [3]. While the management of chronic stable heart

P.T. Campbell, MD (✉)
Heart Transplant Institute, Baptist Health Transplant Institute,
Little Rock, AR, USA
e-mail: Patcamp32@hotmail.com

S. Saberian, MD
Department of Cardiology, University of Illinois College of
Medicine at Peaoria, Peoria, IL, USA

H.O. Ventura (ed.), *Pharmacologic Trends of Heart Failure*,
Current Cardiovascular Therapy,
DOI 10.1007/978-3-319-30593-6_2,
© Springer International Publishing Switzerland 2016

failure has progressed, the management strategies and therapies for ADHF have changed little in the same time period [4]. The mainstay therapies for the management of ADHF are focused on rapidly improving symptoms of dyspnea, peripheral edema and decongesting the patient. Intravenous diuretics are recommended for decongestion and volume removal in all patients with evidence of significant volume overload. Concomitant use of IV vasodilators (nitroprusside, nitroglycerin and neseritide) in patients without evidence of hypotension can aid in decongestion and improve symptoms. In patients with reduced EF and evidence of decreased perfusion and hemodynamic compromise, intravenous inotropes can be used to improve and maintain cardiac output and end-organ perfusion. However none of the therapies have been shown to improve (and may actually increase) morbidity and mortality [5].

The past decade has produced several promising novel therapies for the prevention and treatment acute decompensated heart failure including natriuretic peptides, inotropes and vasodilators.

Modulators of Natriuretic Peptides and Renin Angiotensin Aldosterone System (RAAS)

Vasopeptidase Inhibitors

Vasopeptidase inhibitors (VPIs) are agents that block the activation of the angiotensin converting enzyme (ACE) and neutral endopeptidases simultaneously. ACE, an enzyme that converts angiotensin I into angiotensin II and degrades bradykinin, results in vasoconstriction, along with sodium and water retention. ACE-inhibition decreases the conversion of ANG-I to ANG-II and the degradation of bradykinin. Bradykinin promotes of the vasodilators; NO and prostacyclins [6]. ACE inhibitors are known to improve symptoms, quality of life and reduce hospitalization in the management of patients with congestive heart failure [7]. Neutral endopeptidase (NEP) is an endothelial; membrane-bound metallopeptidase which catalyzes the degradation of vasodilator peptides, including Atrial Natriuretic Peptide (ANP), Brain Natriuretic Peptide (BNP), C-type Natriuretic Peptide (CNP), substance P, and bradykinin [8].These agents act against the Renin-Angiotensin-Aldosterone System (RAAS), cause vasodilation, promote diuresis and natriuresis. NEP acts on both the vasodilatory peptides and simultaneously on vasoconstrictor peptides such as endothelin-1 and ANG-II [8].

Early trials using NEP inhibitors showed mixed results, with certain formulations caused vasoconstriction rather than vasodilation. The effect of NEP inhibition depends on the substrate available, if ANG-II and ET-1 are predominant the NEP inhibitor may result in vasoconstriction, as has been shown in the vasculature of the forearm [9]. Furthermore, the effects of increased natriuretic peptides (ANP) can be attenuated by upregulation of the RAAS and sympathetic nervous system. In clinical trials evaluating the effect of NEP inhibition on vascular tone, Candoxatril showed inconsistent results with no statistically significant benefit in lowering blood pressure compare to placebo [10]. In patients with congestive heart failure, similar results were observed despite noted elevation of ANP and BNP levels [11]. In the advent of ACE inhibitor agents backed by clinical trials, the potential synergistic effects gained from combination of ACE and NEP inhibition created new possibilities in treatment of congestive heart failure by further additional down regulation of the neurohormonal pathways (i.e. sympathetic nervous system and the RAAS pathway).

Earlier trials using Vasopeptidase inhibitors in animal models with hypertension showed significant long lasting effect in reducing the systolic blood pressure in rat models [12]. In hamster models with congestive heart failure, long-term treatment with omapatrilat improved cardiovascular outcomes compared to ACE inhibition with captopril [13]. The early human based trial; the OCTAVE (Omapatrilat and enalapril in patients with hypertension: the Omapatrilat Cardiovascular Treatment vs. Enalapril) trial enrolled 25,000 hypertensive patients who were randomly assigned to either the NEP inhibitor Omapatrilat, or Enalapril. The study demonstrated a greater reduction in systolic blood pressure in the Omapatrilat treatment arm [14]. A smaller study comparing Omapatrilat to Lisinopril found a similar comparison and validated a dose dependent, long lasting effect of Omapatrilat in reduction of blood pressure [15]. In a limited study designed to evaluate the safety and efficacy of a combined NEP-I and ACEI (Sampatrilat) in African American patients with a history of decreased response to ACEI alone, demonstrated improved blood pressure reduction compared to ACEI mono-therapy [16]. The OVERTURE (Omapatrilat Versus Enalapril Randomized Trial of Utility in Reducing Events) trial, which enrolled patients with congestive heart failure (NYHA II–III), demonstrated the beneficial clinical and echocardiographic effects of Vasopeptidase inhibitors. Omapatrilat therapy reduced cardiovascular death by 9 % compared to enalapril, however the primary end-point of death and heart failure hospitalization was not different between the groups [17]. In the IMPRESS trial; a head to head comparison between Omapatrilat and Lisinopril in a randomized control trial, noted that Omapatrilat led to lower incidence of hospitalization and reduction in symptoms while being equally well tolerated within a 12 week period [18].

Despite encouraging results, FDA halted the approval of Vasopeptidase Inhibitors due to the incidence of angioedema in the studied patients. The rate of occurrence was noted to be significantly higher in the OCTAVE trial (2.2 % vs. 0.7 %) compared to ACE inhibitor therapy. The cause of angioedema in patients with ACE inhibition and NEP inhibition was evaluated in select studies and partly attributed to the enzymatic activity of other amino and dipeptidyl peptidases. Further studies suggest the possibility of performing bio testing in order to predict the probability of angioedema prior to treatment [19]. Another factor contributing to lack of approval for NEP inhibitors is a lack of sufficient data in different patient populations; accounting for race, gender, age and medication formulations. Despite shown value in the control of hypertension and clinical benefits in treatment of patient's with congestive heart failure, the risk of unpredictable life threatening angioedema caused a significant set back in the studies and promotion of Vasopeptidase inhibitors.

The concern for severe angioedema was addressed by combining NEP inhibitors with an ARB rather than an ACEI. The angioedema seen in early trials was related to excessive inhibition of the enzymes that degrade bradykinin including ACE and aminopeptidase P. ARB's do not block these enzymes and therefore reduce the risk of life-threatening angioedema. Entresto (sacubitril/valsartan) a neprilysin inhibitor and angiotensin receptor blocker (ARB) combination received FDA approval in July of 2015 after the PARADIGM-HF [20] (Prospective Comparison of ARNI [Angiotensin Receptor – Neprilysin Inhibitor] with ACEI [Angiotensin-Converting–Enzyme Inhibitor to Determine Impact on Global Mortality and Morbidity in Heart Failure) trial was stopped early for overwhelming evidence of benefit over standard ACEI therapy. PARADIGM-HF enrolled primarily NYHA Class II-III FC heart failure patients with elevated BNP levels. Patients were required to have been on prior ACEI or ARB therapy and have an EF <40 %. After 2 years of therapy the NEPI-ARB combination demonstrated significant reductions in the primary composite endpoint of death from cardiovascular causes and heart failure hospitalizations compared to enalapril therapy. The benefit was seen in the individual components as well, it significantly reduced death from cardiovascular causes and demonstrated a 21 % reduction in hospitalization for heart failure. Patients on Entresto had improved functional status, decreased heart failure symptoms and better reported quality of life. The angiotensin-neprilysin inhibitor did have higher rates of symptomatic hypotension and non-serious angioedema, but less cough, renal failure and hyperkalemia.

Sacubitril/valsartan has been approved for the treatment of NYHA Class II–IV heart failure with reduced ejection fraction. The recommended starting dose is 49/51 mg twice daily and can be titrated to a recommended maximum dose of 97/103 mg twice daily. There are recommendations to starting at 24/26 mg twice daily for patients that have severe renal dysfunction, moderate hepatic dysfunction or have never been treated with ACEI/ARB. The significant benefit demonstrated by the PARADIGM-HF study is encouraging for the future of heart failure management. Its full benefits in routine clinical benefits remain to be seen, however ANRI therapy will likely rapidly become standard therapy for the management of chronic heart failure (Table 2.1).

Urodilatin/Ularitide

Natriuretic peptides (NP) have played a large role in the management and understanding of heart failure. Brain-type natriuretic peptide (BNP) and atrial natriuretic peptide (ANP) are released in response to increased myocardial stretch and BNP remains integral in the diagnosis of acute decompensated heart failure (ADHF). Early studies of the recombinant form of BNP (nesiritide) were encouraging, however recent data has failed to demonstrate a significant benefit in the treatment of ADHF [21] and controversy regarding its safety remain [22]. Recent focus has been placed on ANP and its potential therapeutic role in ADHF.

ANP is produced in the atrium primarily in response to increased mycocyte stretch, however ANP can also be released in response to several vasoactive and neurohormones including; epinephrine, vasopression, norepinephrine, angiotensin II and endothelin-1. ANP exerts its biological effects primarily through interaction with the natriuretic peptide receptor type A (NPR-A), the same receptor utilized by BNP. However ANP has up to 70 times the affinity for NPR-A and stimulates ten times greater activity of the NPR-A cyclase [23]. NPR-A receptors are located in a variety of organs and tissues including: vascular smooth muscle, endothelial cells, renal collecting ducts, adrenal glands, kidney, lung, liver and the heart [24, 25]. The binding of ANP to

TABLE 2.1 Summary of clinical trials for neprilysin inhibitors

Study/trial	Aim of study	Dose	Results
Octave	To evaluate the efficacy of Omapatrilat in patients with hypertension, compared to Enalapril	Omapatrilat 10–80 mg, titrated to reach goal BP <140/90 Enalapril 5–40 mg, titrated to reach goal BP <140/90 within 8 weeks, followed for 24 weeks with or without addition of adjuvant therapy to reach target BP goal	Omapatrilat resulted in clinically significant mean reduction of 3–4 mmHg in blood pressure compared to Enalapril Omapatrilat required less up titration of dosage to reach target blood pressure Use of adjuvant therapy post 8 weeks was higher in the Enalapril group Risk of angioedema in the omapatrilat treated patients was (2.17 %) compared to the enalapril treated group (0.68 %) Death and all adverse outcomes were similar between Omapatrilat and Enalapril
Overture	To evaluate the efficacy of Omapatrilat in patients with heart failure (NYHA class II–IV), compared to Enalapril	Enalapril 10 mg twice daily (n – 2884) compared to Omapatrilat 40 mg daily (n – 2886)	No statistically significant reduction in all cause mortality between Omapatrilat, compared to enalapril (hazard ratio 0.94, 95 % confidence interval 0.86–1.03, P = 0.187) Angioedema was more common with Omapatrilat. N = 24 (0.8 %)

(continued)

TABLE 2.1 (continued)

Study/trial	Aim of study	Dose	Results
Impress	To evaluate the efficacy of Omapatrilat on functional capacity and clinical outcomes in patients with heart failure patients, compared to lisinopril	Omapatrilat 40 mg once daily (n – 289) compared to lisinopril 20 mg daily (n – 284) for 24 week	Week 12 exercise treadmill test results improved similarly in the omapatrilat and lisinopril groups (p=0.45) Suggestive trend in favor of omapatrilat on combined endpoints of death or admissions for worsening heart failure (p=0.052; hazard ratio 0.53, 95 % Confidence interval 0.27–1.02) Omapatrilat significantly lowered combined death, admission, or discontinuation of study treatment due worsening heart failure (p=0.035) Omapatrilat improved NYHA class more than lisinopril in patients who had NYHA class III and IV (p=0.035), but not if patients with NYHA class II were included
Paradigm-HF	To evaluate the efficacy of ARB-NEP inhibitor on morbidity and mortality in heart failure patients compared to enalapril	ARB-NEP inhibitor titrated to 200 mg twice daily compared to enalapril titrated to 10 mg twice daily	Significant reduction in combined end-point of death from cardiovascular cause and heart failure hospitalization in the ARB-NEP inhibitor group 21 % (p<0.001) reduction in heart failure hospitalizations with ARB-NEPI Improved symptoms and quality of life in ARB-NEPI group

NPR-A results in increased intracellular concentrations of cGMP [23], resulting in natriuresis, diuresis, vasodilation and inhibition of the renal-angiotensin-aldosterone system (RAAS). In the kidney ANP affects both the renal vasculature and the medullary collecting ducts. ANP-NPR activation in the kidney increases sodium excretion by the collecting ducts enhancing natriuresis and diuresis. ANP acts directly on the renal vasculature vasodilating the afferent and vasoconstricting the efferent arterioles. The increased pressure in the glomerular capillaries results in increased glomerular filtration rate (GFR) [26]. The vasodilatory effects of ANP are mediated through direct increase in cGMP in vascular smooth muscle as well as antagonism of RAAS, vasopressin, epinephrine, endothelin and cytokines [27, 28]. ANP causes equal dilation of both the arterial and venous vasculature and some data suggests that it may have a role in vasodilation of the coronary arteries [24]. The metabolism and removal of ANP is primarily through NPR Type C (clearance) and enzymatic degredation by the neutral endopeptidase (NEP) system. In heart failure the effects of ANP are attenuated compared to healthy individuals even in the setting of increased circulating levels. Theories the attenuated effect of ANP in chronic heart failure include: chronic upregulation of ANP production results in the release of less biologically active molecules [29], downregulation of NPR-A receptors and increased NEP activity [30].

Carperitide is a recombinant form of ANP, currently approved in Japan for the treatment of ADHF. A small randomized controlled study (PROTECT) reported significant reductions in death and rehospitalization in patients with reduced EF (<35 %) treated with Carperitide [31], however large scale trials confirming these outcomes are lacking. The hemodynamic benefits of Carperitide are unclear, one study [32] failed to demonstrate improved hemodynamics (PCWP, RAP) with Carperitide compared to traditional intravenous vasodilators, while a more recent study [33] reported improved hemodynamic parameters compared with vasodilator therapy. The conflicting data regarding the hemodynamic benefits of Carpertide may be due to increased degradation of ANP by the NEP system or the down regulation of NPR-A receptors in chronic heart failure. The two largest observational studies of Carperitide for the treatment of ADHF [34, 35] demonstrated similar results. Caperitide improved dyspnea scores in younger patients (<65 years) with Heart Failure with preserved EF (HFpEF) and mild/moderate decompensation without acute ischemia. The most common adverse event was hypotension, which occurred in 5–10 % of patients. Carperitide was less effective and caused significantly more hypotension in older patients, patients with acute myocardial ischemia and reduced renal function. The limited data regarding Carperitide seems to suggest a possible role in the treatment of patients with ADHF in the setting of hypertensive heart disease and/or HFpEF. Larger studies and more robust data are required before Caperitide can be recommended for routine treatment of ADHF.

Urodilatin is a modified pro-ANP produced in the kidneys, first osilated from human urine [36]. Urodilation binds to NPR-A receptors with equal affinity as ANP, and exerts similar hemodynamic effects as intravenous ANP [25]. Urodilatin differs slightly from ANP in molecular confirmation, which confers resistance to NEP degradation. Early studies of urodilantin demonstrated similar yet sustained hemodynamic effects compared to ANP, suggesting prolonged activity may be due to its resistance to NEP degradation [37]. Ularitide is a synthetic form of Urodilatin that has shown promising results in the management of ADHF. Animal studies demonstrated improved hemodynamic, natriuretic and diuretic effects from Ularitide administration. Early trials in patients with ADHF, both bolus [37] and infusions [38] of Ularitide resulted in decreases in PCWP, systemic vascular resistance and right atrial pressure (RAP). Ularitide favorably affected natriuresis and diuresis. Results from SIRIUS I, a pilot trial [39] demonstrated significant improvement in dyspnea and hemodynamics when Ularitide was added to standard HF therapy including diuretics. There was no difference in urine output between the ularitide and placebo groups, however the

Ularitide group received less frequent and lower doses of diuretics. The hemodynamic and possible diuretic benefits of Ularitide occurred without negative impact on renal function. Hypotension occurred in almost 17 % of the treatment group without impact on clinical outcomes. The highest dose of Ularitide was associated with greater hemodynamic benefits, but resulted in significantly greater hypotension (−17 mmHg in SBP). The follow-up, larger randomized SIRIUS II trial [40] confirm the results of SIRIUS I. Ularitide resulted in favorable reductions in PCWP, right atrial pressure (RAP), systemic vascular resistance (SVR) and improved dyspnea. The effects of ularitide were observed throughout the entire 24 h of infusion without deleterious effects on short-term outcome. An important finding in the SIRIUS II trial was a dose dependent decline in myocardial oxygen consumption in the treatment group. Further analysis of the SIRIUS II [41] data revealed the potential renal protective effects of the intermediate dose (15 ng/kg/min) of Ularitide in HF patients. Ularitide resulted in a favorable effect on the MAP-RAP pressure gradient (an estimate of renal perfusion) which improved renal perfusion and may have contributed to short-term preservation of renal function. Ularitide resulted in sustained MAP while simultaneously reducing RAP. Similar results were not observed in the highest dose, likely due to more substantial reductions in MAP. In patients with ADHF infusions of Ularitide seem to improve hemodynamic parameters, antagonize neurohormonal activity, improve diuresis, preserve renal function and reduce myocardial oxygen demand, however long-term clinical benefits have yet to be demonstrated. Ularitide has not be approved for routine use, however data from the SIRIUS trials suggest that the intermediate dose of 15 ng/kg/min may provide the desired benefits while potentially limiting the incidence and severity of hypotension. With concern regarding the efficacy and safety of other natriuretic peptides, the ultimate role of Ularitide in the treatment of heart failure remains to be seen. Future studies randomized trials are required to assess the long-term risk and benefits associated with natriuretic peptide therapy.

Vasodilator Therapies

Relaxin

Relaxin is a naturally occurring peptide that was first isolated from pregnant guinea pigs and rabbits [42] and later found to have cardiovascular effects including; increased cardiac output, increased arterial compliance and reduced SVR, along with increased renal blood flow, during human pregnancy [43]. Relaxin acts on multiple pathways with possible vasodilatory, angiogenesis and anti-inflammatory effects (Fig. 2.1). Relaxin exerts the majority of its effects through a g-protein coupled receptor, LGR-7, which has been isolated in human systemic vascular, renal vascular and cardiac tissues [46]. Relaxin acts

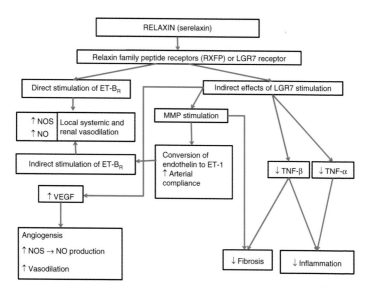

FIGURE 2.1 Effect of Relaxin Receptor activation by Serelaxin. Notes: *ET-BR* endothelin-B receptor, *NOS* nitric oxide synthase, *NO* nitric oxide, *MMP* matrix metalloproteinase, *VEGF* vascular endothelial growth factor, *TNF* tumor necrosis factor. (Adapted from Teichman [44] and Teichman [45])

through multiple pathways that ultimately result in increased nitric oxide (NO) production and vasodilation. One of the predominant pathways utilized by Relaxin is the endothelin system. The endothelin system comprises two major receptors, Endothelin-A (ET-A) receptors and Endothelin-B (ET-B) receptors. ET-A is responsible for vasoconstriction, while ET-B is primarily responsible for vasodilation in the vascular system. Relaxin has been shown to act both directly and indirectly on the ET system and may increase ET-B receptor expression [47]. The Relaxin-LGR-7 (RLX-7) ligand acts primarily by stimulating matrix metalloproteins 2 and 9 (MMP) which convert Endothelin (ET) into active ET_{1-32}. The activated ET_{1-32} bind to ET-B receptors which then increase NO production and result in vasoldilation. The increased NO production results in vasodilation of both the systemic and renal vasculature. In the systemic vasculature the RLX-7 ligand can also directly activate the ET-B receptor resulting in increased NO production. There is evidence that RLX-7 increases local phosphatidylinositol 3-kinase and NO resulting in rapid vasodilation [48]. In the kidneys the RLX-7 ligand inhibits the Na/K+ ATPase, which may be the mechanism of the observed natriuresis and diuresis.

Few randomized clinical trials evaluating the efficacy and safety of relaxin for the management of heart failure have been published. The Pre-RELAX-AHF was a small, randomized pilot study that evaluated a 48 h infusion of escalating doses of Relaxin compared to placebo for the treatment of acute decompensated heart failure and mild to moderate renal dysfunction. The study demonstrated reductions in the composite endpoint of cardiovascular mortality, heart failure hospitalization or hospitalization for renal failure [49].

The larger RELAX-AHF study enrolled 1161 patients with acute decompensated heart failure with evidence of congestion (pulmonary congestion on chest x-ray and elevated BNP) and mild to moderate renal dysfunction (GFR 30–75 mL/min/m²). Patients were randomized to a 48 h infusion of Serelaxin (30 μg/kg/day) versus placebo. Patients with SBP <125 mmHg were excluded from the trial.

The administration of serealxin resulted in significant declines in early worsening of heart failure, overall length of stay and ICU length of stay. The treatment group reported significantly greater mild reduction in dyspnea and earlier improvement in symptoms. There was a 37 % reduction in cardiovascular and all-cause mortality, however the study was not powered to assess mortality. Serelaxin was associated with greater rates of clinically significant hypotension requiring dose adjustment but less worsening renal function [50]. The major criticism of the RELAX-AHF trial was the generalizability of the data to the larger heart failure population. Patients in the study had significantly higher BP compared to most heart failure studies, almost half of the patients had ejection fraction >40 % and the vast majority (95 %) were Caucasian. While symptomatic improvement is important for the treatment of patients with ADHF, future studies are required to determine if the signal for improved mortality seen is real.

Inotropic Agents

Istaroxime

Istaroxime (Istaroxime-(E,Z)-3-[(2-aminoethoxy)-imino] androstane-6,17-dione is a novel drug with dual action that while unrelated to cardiac glycosides (digoxin) shares one similar mechanism of action. Istaroxime inhibits the Na+/K+ ATPase and simultaneously stimulates the sarcoplasmic endoplasmic reticulum calcium ATPase isoform 2 (SERCA2a), thereby affecting both myocyte contraction and relaxation [51]. The inhibition of Na+/K+ ATPase results in increased cytosolic calcium concentrations during diastole and intracellular Ca2+ concentrations is essential for sarcomere shortening and cardiac myocyte contractions. SERCA2a stimulation results in rapid reuptake of Ca2+ into the sarcoplasmic reticulum (SR) during diastole and enhances myocyte relaxation and lusitropy. The efficient uptake of Ca2+

into the SR also results in sufficient SR Ca2+ concentrations to facilitate subsequent cardiac contractions.

In the heart, calcium cycling is responsible for triggering the interaction between actin and myosin, which result in cardiac contraction. During systole, an action potential stimulates the influx of Ca2+ through L-type Ca2+ channels and the increase in intracellular Ca2+ induces release of Ca2+ from the SR through ryanodine receptor (RyR2) channels. The increased intracellular Ca2+ concentrations is responsible for the contraction of cardiac myocytes [52]. During diastole the RyR2 channels close, the Ca2+ dissociates from the myofilaments and intracellular Ca2+ decline. The rapid decline in intracellular Ca2+ concentrations result in myocardial relaxation, also referred to as lusitropy. There are three mechanisms by which the intracellular Ca2+ concentrations are decreased during diastole, the first is through rapid reuptake of Ca2+ into the SR by SERCA2a, which accounts for approximately 70 %. SERCA2a activity is modulated by phosphorylation of phospholamban (PLB), if unphosphorylated it inhibits the activity of SERCA, while phosphorylated phopholamban activates SERCA. Thus phosphorylated PLB is integral to lusitropy. The second is through the Na+/Ca2+ Exchanger (NCX), which moves Ca2+ extracellularly and is responsible for approximately 28 % of the Ca2+ reuptake. The final mechanism is through the plasma membrane Ca2+ ATPase [51, 53].

In the heterogeneity of heart failure calcium dysregulation has been demonstrated to play a role in certain etiologies. Calcium "leak" from the SR during diastole due to abnormal RyR2 channels has been demonstrated. This "leak" results in decreased Ca2+ availability during systole which decreases the contractile force generated by the myocytes [54]. Abnormal function of the SERCA2a pump has also been shown to impact both contraction and relaxation of the cardiac myocyte. Reduced SERCA activity results in decreased reuptake into the SR which results in creased concentrations of Ca2+ available during systole and sustained levels of intracellular Ca2+ during diastole results in decreased relaxation and diastolic dysfunction [55]. Finally reduced phosphorylation of the PLB protein may also alter the efficiency of SERCA2a in heart failure, affecting both lusitropy and inotropy [56]. Istaroxime may improve cardiac calcium cycling thereby improving relaxation, contraction and the oxygen demand of the cardiac myocyte. In the mechanically challenged heart the reduction of SERCA2a activity results in upregulation of the NCX channels, extracellular exchange of $Ca2+$ for $Na+$. The increased NCX activity results in slower reduction of intracellular $Ca2+$ concentrations, negatively impacting cardiac relaxation and reducing the available $Ca2+$ for systole [57]. Furthermore it results in increased energy demands, the NCX pathway requires twice as much energy as the SERCA channels and requires increased $Na+/K+$ ATPase activity to maintain intracellular $Na+$ levels, all at an increased energy cost to the strained mycocardium [58].

Istaroxime has dual activity in the cardiac myocyte, it inhibits the $Na+/K+$ ATPase, which results in increased cytoplasmic concentrations of $Ca2+$ and simultaneously stimulates SERCA2a affinity for $Ca2+$. The increased SERCA2a activity improves both cardiac relaxation and contraction. The combined activity of Istaroxime, increasing systolic intracellular $Ca2+$ concentration and rapid sequestration of $Ca2+$ during diastole, result in both increased contractility and improved diastolic function. Early animal studies with Istaroxime resulted in improved inotropy and lusitropy. In a hamster model of dilated cardiomyopathy, long-term oral administration demonstrated mortality benefits [59]. The positive inotropic and lusitropic were observed without significant side-effects including arrhythmia, heart rate, blood pressure or myocardial oxygen demand. In a second animal study [60] similar beneficial effects of Istaroxime were demonstrated in hemodynamic and echocardiographic parameters in dogs. Dose-dependent improvement was seen in left ventricular ejection fraction (LVEF), End-diastolic pressures (LVEDP), end-diastolic (EDV), end-systolic volumes (ESV), stroke volume (SV), coronary blood flow (CBF) and deceleration time (DT). The hemodynamic improvements were obtained without significant increases in myocardial oxygen consumption.

The HORIZON-HF was a large randomized, double-blind, placebo controlled study evaluating the effects of Istaroxime in patients admitted for decompensated heart failure with reduced ejection fraction (HFrEF) [61, 62]. The study included 120 patients between 18 and 85 years of age with reduced EF (<35 %) and a pulmonary capillary wedge pressure (PCWP) >20 mmHg on invasive hemodynamic assessment.. Patients were randomized to an infusion of 0.5, 1.0, 1.5 µg/kg/min of Istaroxime or placebo for 6 h. The primary endpoint was change in pulmonary capillary wedge pressure (PCWP) after 6 h infusion. Secondary endpoints included change in cardiac index (CI), right atrial pressure (RAP), systolic BP, diastolic BP, heart rate (HR), along with echocardiographic assessment of systolic and diastolic function. Other parameters assessed included neurohormones, renal function, and troponin. After the 6 h infusion Istaroxime significantly reduced PCWP compared to placebo in a dose dependent manner for all three doses. The greatest decline in PCWP (–4.7 mmHg) was observed in the 1.5 µg/kg/min dose compared to no change in the placebo group. Istaroxime also significantly increased SBP in the highest dose by 15 mmHg compared placebo. During infusion of the highest dose, Istaroxime improved cardiac index (CI) but was not significant at 6 h. Istaroxime improved regional and global myocardial systolic and diastolic function, and LV compliance as assessed by tissue-doppler echocardiography.

The improved PCWP and diastolic function were observed without significant adverse events, changes in neurohormones or increase in troponin. The lack of increase in troponin suggest that the inotropic and lusitropic effects of Istaroxime occurred without significant increase in myocardial oxygen consumption, these findings are consistent with the findings in the animal studies. The only significant adverse events noted were nausea, vomiting and injection site pain.

The data from current available evidence suggest Istaroxime may provide beneficial effects in patients with ADHF, without significant adverse effects. The combination of increased SERCA2a activity and inhibition of the Na+/K+ ATPase channels results in improved energy balance, decreasing the myocardial oxygen consumption in the failing heart. The increased affinity of SERCA for Ca2+ improves both myocardial relaxation by increasing the rapid reuptake into the SR and improves myocardial contraction through increased availability of Ca2+. The data seems to suggest that Istaroxime improves cardiac Ca2+ cycling and increases intracellular Ca2+ concentrations without the risk of increased arrhythmogenesis [63]. In fact the HORIZON-HF study demonstrated a significant shortening of the QTc in patients treated with Istaroxime [61].

Although not currently FDA approved, recent literature suggest that Istaroxime may be beneficial in patients admitted for acute decompensated heart failure (NYHA Class II–III) with reduced LVEF. Data from the HORIZON-HF suggest doses between 0.5 and 1.5 μg/kg/min may be useful for the management of ADHF. Istaroxime has a 1 h half-life and reached steady state levels at 4 h after of infusion. Istaroxime is metabolized to three less active metabolites and is not excreted by the kidneys [61]. While the most benefit was seen in the highest dose, adverse events were more common at that dose. Future studies focused on in-hospital and long-term clinical outcomes are required to determine the future of this promising drug.

Levosimendan

Commonly used agents in patients with acute decompensated heart failure with systolic dysfunction are intravenous inotropic agents, of which B-adrenergic agonists and phosphodiesterase inhibitors encompass the majority. β-adrenergic agents augment the release calcium into the myocytes by increasing intracellular cAMP levels. Phosphodiesterase inhibitors perform a similar task by inhibiting the degradation of cAMP [64]. Increased intracellular calcium increases contractility, but is also associated with increased risk of arrhythmia and mortality [65]. Levosimendan is a new agent, which acts by sensitizing cardiac troponin C to calcium. This unique mechanism of action strengthens contraction without increasing oxygen demand, cAMP or intracellular calcium concentrations [66]. Levosimendan functions by binding to the regulatory domain and the charged amino acids in the hydrophobic pocket of the calcium saturated N-terminal domain of the troponin C [67]. In a calcium dependent manner, Levosimendan stabilizes the conformation of calcium–troponin C complex through hydrophobic and electrostatic interactions. This results in accelerated actin–myosin cross bridge formation rate and reduces the speed of dissociation [68]. Levosimendan has also been shown to improve both peripheral and coronary vasodilation. The afterload reduction likely contributes to its effectiveness and the coronary vasodilation may improve cardiac myocyte oxygen mismatch [69].

The effect of Levosimendan is attenuated during diastole due to reduced intracellular Ca2+ concentrations as a result of active Ca2+ reuptake. This allows for appropriate left ventricular relaxation, while maintaining its inotropic properties during the systolic phase of the cardiac cycle [70]. Outside the cardiac myocyte Levosimendan stimulates ATP-dependent potassium channels in myocytes and vascular smooth muscle cells, resulting in vasodilatation [71]. Levosimendan is generally well tolerated in all clinical trials to date. The most frequent adverse effect is headache, hypotension, dizziness and nausea. These side effects are largely attributed to the vasodilatory effect of Levosimendan. Decrease in hemoglobin and hematocrit in higher doses have been reported, as well a mild hypokalemia without significant clinical outcomes.

Levosimendan is an infusion agent with a rapid onset of action, a short half-life of 1.3 h and an active metabolite known as OR-1986 [72]. OR-1986 is formed by the acetylation of Levosimendan metabolites formed by colonic bacteria upon its secretion. It is less plasma bound than its native parent and thus more potent. The peak concentration of OR-1896 is reached within 2–3 days post infusion and its effects may persist for 7–9 days [73]. The initial dosing recommended based on clinical trial is a bolus infusion of 6–12 µg/kg over 10 min, followed by a maintenance dose of 0.05–0.2 µg/kg/min over 24–48 h [74].

Several studies have evaluated the safety, efficacy and hemodynamic outcomes of Levosimendan in humans. An early randomized clinical trial in 146 patients with heart failure NYHA class III–IV, with known cardiac index of

<2.5 L/min/m^2 and elevated wedge pressure (PCWP) showed favorable results. This study concluded that Levosimendan was associated with a dose dependent increase in stroke volume and cardiac index and decrease in PCWP at various doses [75]. Clinical symptoms of dyspnea and fatigue were also improved without any clinical adverse effects. The LIDO (Levosimendan Infusion vs Dobutamine in Severe Low Output Heart Failure) study compared the effect of Levosimendan to Dobutamine. It was found that a significantly higher proportion of Levosimendan patients showed improved cardiac output ($\geq 30\%$ increase) and a concomitant decrease in PCWP ($\geq 25\%$). It was also found that 180-day mortality was lower in the Levosimendan subgroup [76].

The CASINO (Calcium Sensitizer or Inotrope or None in Low Output Heart Failure Study) trial, patients with NYHA-IV classification and reduced left ventricular function showed statistically significant reduction in mortality in a 6-month period compared to patients treated with Dobutamine [77]. From a mortality perspective, The SURVIVE study evaluated 1327 hospitalized patients with acute decompensated heart failure found early benefits from the use of Levosimendan but no difference in mortality and incidence of adverse effects [78]. The REVIVE II study; which evaluated 600 patients with acute decompensated heart failure, demonstrated that Levosimendan in addition to standard therapy was superior to standard therapy alone and resulted in a shorter duration of hospitalization. There was no significant difference in 90-day mortality and concerns were raised regarding an increased rate of arrhythmias [79].

Use of Levosimendan in patients with cardiogenic shock has shown favorable results in those treated in conjugation with catecholamines for restoration of hemodynamics. While studied in a small sample size, Levosimendan treatment resulted in a significant increase in cardiac output together with a decrease in systemic vascular resistance and decreased mortality at 6 months [80, 81]. The RUSSLAN (Randomized Study on Safety and Effectiveness of Levosimendan in Patients with Left Ventricular Failure due to an Acute Myocardial Infarction) trial evaluated 504 patients with reduced left ventricular ejection fraction due to recent myocardial infarction. Use of Levosimendan was associated with decrease in mortality and worsening heart failure compared with placebo at 6 and 24 h after the infusion with lower all-cause mortality at 14 days in the treatment group. This lower mortality persisted at 180 days but without a statistically significance [82]. On going large clinical trials including the LION-Heart, LAICA and ELEVATE are underway evaluating the role intermittent dosing of Levosimendan in overall mortality and hospitalization rate.

Major contraindications to Levosimendan include moderate to severe renal impairment, severe hepatic impairment, ventricular filling and outflow obstruction, hypotension, tachycardia and a history of Torsades de pointes. No dose change is required for mild renal or hepatic insufficiency. Levosimendan is administered as loading dose of 6–12 μg/kg over 10 min. It is followed by infusion 0.05–0.2 mcg/kg/min for up to 24 h. Levosimendan administration has been well tolerated when co-administered with standard heart failure therapies; ACE inhibitor, B-blockers, Isosorbite mononitrate, warfarin and digoxin, without significant drug-drug interactions [83]. The European society of cardiology recommends against the use of Levosimendan in patients with significant hypotension (SBP < 85 mmHg). Use of Levosimendan is not yet approved by the FDA. Levosimendan has since been approved by many European countries and used when indicated. Current clinical trails have largely been conducted in European countries. Evidence supporting the role of Levosimendan in improving and restoration of hemodynamics in patients with decompensated heart failure are many. Its role in reduction of mortality in long term follow up and appropriate intermittent dosing are current topics in ongoing clinical trials (Table 2.2).

Table 2.2 Summary of Levosimendan clinical trials

Study/study	Aim	Dose	Results
LIDO	To evaluate the effects of Levosimendan on hemodynamic performance and clinical outcomes in heart failure patients, compared to Dobutamine	103 patients assigned to Levosimendan and given an infusion of 24 µg/kg over 10 min, followed by a continuous infusion of 0.1 µg/kg/min for 24 h. 100 patients assigned to Dobutamine and infused for 24 h at an initial dose of 5 µg/kg/min	The primary hemodynamic endpoint (30 % increase in cardiac output or 25 % decrease in pulmonary capillary wedge pressure) was achieved in 29 (28 %) Levosimendan-group patients and 15 (15 %) in the Dobutamine group (hazard ratio 1.9, 95 % Confidence interval 1.1–3.3, p=0.022)
			At 180 days, 27 (26 %) Levosimendan-group patients had died, compared with 38 (38 %) in the Dobutamine group (hazard ratio 0.57, CI 0.34–0.95, p=0.029) Both Levosimendan and Dobutamine increased heart rate by a modest and similar amount
			Renal and Liver dysfunction declined in the Levosimendan group
			Clinical symptoms of dyspnea and fatigue improved more so with Levosimendan, however not statistically significant

CASINO   To evaluate the efficacy of Levosimendan on composite of death or re-hospitalization in heart failure patients compared to placebo or Dobutamine

299 patients with decompensated heart failure (Ejection fraction <35 %) receiving 24 h infusion of Levosimendan, placebo or Dobutamine

The study was designed to recruit 600 patients, but it was stopped after 299 patients had been recruited due to clear superiority of Levosimendan versus placebo or Dobutamine
6 months mortality was 18 % in the Levosimendan treatment group, 42 % in the Dobutamine group and 28.3 % for placebo

SURVIVE To evaluate the effect of Levosimendan on clinical outcomes in patients with heart failure compared to Dobutamine

1327 patients with heart failure (Ejection fraction <30 %) receiving Levosimendan (n – 664) with bolus dose of 12 μg/kg followed by dose increase of 0.1–0.2/kg/min for 24 h or Dobutamine (n – 663) with a continuous dose of 5 μg/kg/min

Mortality rates in patients treated with Levosimendan was not significantly superior to Dobutamine (26 vs. 28 %, respectively, Hazard ratio 0.91 (95 % Confidence interval 0.74–1.13, $P = 0.401$)
Levosimendan use was attributed to higher rates of Atrial Fibrillation compared to Dobutamine (9.1 % vs. 6.1 %)
Levosimendan use was associated with lower incidence of heart failure worsening (12.3 % vs. 17 %) compared with Dobutamine
Incidence of hypotension and ventricular arrhythmias were similar

(continued)

Table 2.2 (continued)

Study/study	Aim	Dose	Results
REVIVE II	To evaluate the effect of Levosimendan on Clinical outcomes in patients with heart failure as adjuvant therapy to standard therapy	600 patients with heart failure (Ejection fraction <30 %) receiving Levosimendan with bolus dose of 12 µg/kg followed by dose increase of 0.1–0.2 µg/kg/min for 24 h. Patients were followed for up to 4 days post infusion completion	Levosimendan treatment was associated with improved outcomes (19.4 % experienced improvement in clinical findings vs. 14.6 % in placebo, p=0.015), Levosimendan use was associated with decrease in duration of hospitalization by approximately 2 days ((7.9 vs. 8.9 days in placebo, p=0.001) No significant reduction in mortality was observed within the follow up period Levosimendan use was associated with higher incidence of hypotension (50 % vs. 36 %), Ventricular Arrhythmias (25 % vs. 17 %) and Atrial Fibrillation (8 % vs. 2 %) compared to placebo

RUSSLAN	To evaluate the effect of Levosimendan on clinical outcomes in patients with left ventricular failure due to as acute myocardial infarction	504 patients treated with Levosimendan with four different loading doses (0.1–0.4 μg/kg/min) for 6 h compared to placebo	The incidence of ischemia with or without hypotension was similar in all treatment groups (P=0.319) An increase in Incidence of myocardial ischemia and/or hypotension was seen in the highest Levosimendan dose group Levosimendan was associated with lower risk of death and worsening heart failure, compared to placebo during the 6 h infusion (2.0 % vs. 5.9 %; P=0.033) and over 24 h (4.0 % vs. 8.8 %; P=0.044) Levosimendan was noted for decreased mortality compared with placebo at 14 days (11.7 % vs. 19.6 %, hazard ratio 0.56, 95 % CI 0.33–0.95, P=0.031) and the reduction was maintained at the 180-day retrospective follow-up (22.6 % vs. 31.4 %, Hazard ratio 0.67, 95 % confidence interval 0.45–1.00, P=0.053)

Omecamtiv Mecarbil

Myocardial contraction by the sarcomeres within the myocytes is initiated through the transduction of chemical into
mechanical energy. The force generating structures within the
sarcomeres consist of actin and myosin, which are regulated
by regulatory proteins troponin and tropomyosin. Each myosin complex consists of two myosin heavy chains and two
light chains. Each myosin heavy chain head consists of an
ATPase complex that cleaves ATP to produce energy, as well
as an actin-binding site. Cardiac troponin and tropomyosin
form a complex that regulates the interaction of myosin with
actin in a calcium dependent process [84]. Increased calcium
concentration via depolarization of the myocytes causes
binding of calcium to cardiac troponin and dissociation of the
troponin-tropomyosin complex. This process allows for actin-
myosin cross bridge formation and hydrolysis of ATP to
ADP + Pi. The subsequent release of the Pi results in bending
of the myosin head, producing a 10-nm stroke. Calcium is
then stored in the sarcoplasmic reticulum waiting for the next
cycle of myocardial activation. The actin-myosin cycle is
quintessential in generation of the myocardial force and contractility [85]. The current drugs that influence the cardiac
contractility act by increasing intracellular cAMP and
Calcium. These agents have been associated with hypotension and increased myocardial demand due to the increased
myocardial oxygen demand. These agents, in the setting of
ongoing myocardial ischemia and decompensated heart failure, are associated with increased risk of arrhythmias and
mortality [86].

Omecamtiv Mecarbil, known as CK-1827452, is the fourth
candidate compound produced which increases the cardiac
myosin ATpase activity but not other muscle myosins. It has
a half-life that ranges from 17.1 to 21 h. It is the only compound of its class that was studied in human populations and
is considered the successor to previous models that showed
favorable results in animal models only [87]. Omecamtiv
Mecarbil functions by improving energy mobilization and

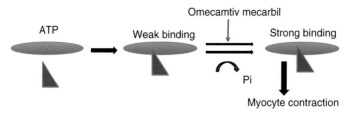

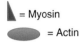

FIGURE 2.2 Mechanism of action: Omecamtiv Mecarbil. *Pi* phosphate (The mechanism of action of Omecamtiv Mecarbil; increasing rate of strong binding through increased rate of phosphate release from myosin, which is the rate limiting step of myocyte activation)

enhancing the myosin-actin cross bridge formation and duration [88]. It also facilitates the release of the phosphate group from myosin heads; thereby increasing the time spent contracting without altering the velocity of the contraction [89]. Omecamtiv Mecarbil increases the rate of transition from weakly bound myosin-actin filaments to the strongly bound state, which enables the myocyte contraction (Fig. 2.2). There are no changes in calcium concentrations within the sarcoplasmic reticulum or the calcium made available for each cycle [90]. Earlier animal studies in rat and dog models with left ventricular hypertrophy and heart failure, utilizing Omecamtiv Mecarbil showed a 20 % increase in left ventricular ejection fraction, systolic time, systolic wall thickening and stroke volume [91]. Interestingly, the studies also showed a reduction in left ventricular end diastolic pressure, mean left atrial pressure and heart rate with no changes in blood flow to the endocardium and myocardial oxygen demand.

In the first human study with Omecamtiv Mecarbil, 34 patients were randomized and received 6-h infusions weekly for 4 weeks. Echocardiograms were obtained prior and post administration of infusions. Researchers found a linear dose dependent increase in left ventricular systolic time and statistically significant changes in ejection fraction and fractional shortening [92]. Doses that were well tolerated were infusions at 0.625 mg/kg/h and below. Patients receiving higher doses developed signs and symptoms of myocardial ischemia due to severe prolongation of the systolic ejection time, thereby decreasing the diastolic time and coronary perfusion. A second randomized clinical trial evaluated 45 patients with known heart failure with ejection fraction <40 %. This study concluded that Omecamtiv Mecarbil was associated with improved systolic ejection time, stroke volume and fractional shortening in a concentration dependent manner with no changes in the E/E′ or S′ [93]. Three patients were found to have elevated cardiac biomarkers out of the 151 infusions during this study. Two patients showed sign and symptoms of myocardial ischemia; one due to accidental overdose while the other was attributed to poor mechanisms of clearance and therefore increased plasma concentrations beyond predicted values. A phase II clinical trial that evaluated the role of Omecamtiv Mecarbil on patients with ischemic cardiomyopathy found no clinically significant deleterious effect in patients with serum concentrations that improved cardiac function [94]. The ATOMIC-AHF trial randomized 613 patients with left ventricular systolic dysfunction who were admitted for worsening dyspnea. This study showed no significant benefit at lower serum concentrations in improving symptoms. Although the study did not reach clinical significance in the primary end-point, there was improved dyspnea in patients on the highest dose of omecamtiv mecarbil. Interestingly there were also signals of decreases in worsening heart failure and ventricular arrhythmias [95].

Omecamtiv Mecarbil has shown a dose and concentration dependent effect on cardiac function. The recommended initial infusion dosing based on early human studies was 0.125 mg/kg/h; in which increase in systolic ejection time, fractional shortening and stroke volume are noted. Doses up to 0.625 mg/kg/h were well tolerated during studies.

Improvement in ejection fraction was noted at doses of 0.5 mg/kg/h or greater. Adverse outcomes were attributed to plasma concentrations exceeding 1200 ng/mL and were universally attributed to decreased diastolic filling time and coronary perfusion. All research thus far in evaluating the pharmacokinetics and effect of Omecamtiv Mecarbil has provided guidelines for appropriate dosing selection and monitoring for future trials. The role of Omecamtiv Mecarbil in patients with acute decompensated heart failure with NYHA III–IV with inadequate cardiac output remains under evaluated with no answer in sight with regards to clinical effects on quality of life, morbidity and mortality. Required IV infusions and serum concentration monitoring may represent further challenges. Having established grounds regarding appropriate dosing, concentration monitoring, tolerability, and improved cardiac function, further studies are warranted in the evaluation of this novel agent in the management of decompensated heart failure with reduced ejection fraction.

Adjunctive Therapies

Tolvaptan

Vasopressin is a 9 amino acid peptide, which is produced by the magnocellular neurosecretory cells of the supraoptic nucleus and the paraventricular nucleus of the hypothalamus. It is stored in the posterior pituitary and secreted into the systemic circulation [96]. The release of Vasopressin is primarily driven by changes in serum osmolality as detected by specialized sensors in the brain, and changes in circulating blood volume as perceived by baroreceptors in the carotid sinus, the atria, pulmonary trunk and stretch receptors in large veins [97, 98]. Vasopressin functions by acting on the cells within the collecting ducts of the kidneys, where the insertion of unique water channels (called aquaporin 2) into the luminal membrane allow for free water reabsorption into the systemic circulation [99]. Vasopressin receptors are

G-protein receptors of which three types are known, V_1, V_2 and V_{1B}. V_1 receptors are abundant in vascular smooth muscles and cause vasoconstriction upon activation. V_2 receptors mediate the antidiuretic response in the collecting ducts of the renal tubules while the V_{1B} receptors in the anterior pituitary mediate the release of adrenocorticotropic hormone and endorphins [100, 101].

Tolvaptan is an oral Vasopressin antagonist first described in 1998 [102] and approved by the FDA in 2009 for the treatment of hypervolumic or euvolumic hypotonic hyponatremia (Defined as serum sodium <125 mEq/L or less marked hyponatremia that is symptomatic and has persisted despite adequate volume restriction). Tolvaptan antagonizes the V_1 and V_2 receptors, thereby preventing free water reabsorption. It binds V_2 receptors with an affinity 1.8 times greater than inherent Vasopressin and 29 times greater than V_1. Tolvaptan has a half-life of approximately 9.4 h. It is plasma protein bound with a peak concentration of 2 h with no alteration in effect by food intake [103]. The majority of the metabolism occurs in the liver through the CYP3A4/5 enzymatic mediated process, while a small fraction of its clearance is medicated by the renal system. Vasopressin is primarily released in response to a hypovolemia and hypotension. In a seemingly paradoxical response vasopressin levels are not suppressed and may even be elevated in heart failure. The up regulation of vasopressin in heart failure results in increased vasoconstriction, increased salt and fluid retention. These effects are similar to the effects seen as a result of the up regulation of the RAAS system, which has been associated with a poor prognosis in patients with known systolic dysfunction via retention of free water and resulting hyponatremia [104].

The SALT-1 and SALT-2 trials were the initial large randomized clinical trials, which evaluated the effect of Tolvaptan on euvolemic and hypervolemic, hyponatremic patients. Heart failure patients comprised 33 and 29 % of enrolled patients in the SALT-1, and 29 % in the SALT-2 trial, respectively [105]. Both trials concluded that Tolvaptan could be safely administered in a 30-day period to increase serum NA^+ concentrations through removal of excess free water. The role of Tolvaptan in heart failure patients has been analyzed in many clinical trials. Early randomized studies in patients with heart failure symptoms showed weight reduction and normalization of sodium concentrations without amendments in quality of life, reduction of systolic or diastolic blood pressures or negative impact on renal function [106]. The ACTIV in CHF (Acute and Chronic Therapeutic Impact of Vasopressin Antagonist in Congestive Heart Failure) trial studied the effect of Tolvaptan in hospitalized individuals with known LV dysfunction who presented with worsening symptoms of their heart failure. Gheorghiade M et al. showed a statistically significant reduction in weight and dyspnea in the treatment group compared to placebo in a short-term analysis (up to 10 days) with no significant difference in worsening HF between the two groups during the outpatient follow up period of the study [107]. The EVEREST (Efficacy of Vasopresin Antagonism in Heart Failure Outcome Study With Tolvaptan) trial randomized 4133 patients presenting with HF symptoms and reduced EF to either tolvaptan or placebo. The authors found improvements in dyspnea, weight loss and edema in the treatment group. Importantly these benefits occurred without significantly higher incidence of adverse events including hypotension, hypernatremia or renal failure [108]. The ECLIPSE (Effect of tolvaptan on hemodynamic Parameters in Subjects with Heart Failure) trial analyzed the hemodynamic effect of Tolvaptan in heart failure patients with NYHA III & IV. It concluded that no significant changes in cardiac index, pulmonary vascular resistance, and systemic vascular resistance were noted in the treatment group while a statistically significant decrease in peak change in PCWP was noted from 3 to 8 h after Tolvaptan administration [109]. The METEOR (Multicenter, randomized, double-blind, placebo-controlled study on the effect of oral tolvaptan on left ventricular dilation and function in patients with heart failure and systolic dysfunction) study subsequently failed to show a significant change in LV ejection fraction post 1 year of therapy with Tolvaptan 30 mg/daily in 240 patients with LV function <30 % [110].

While trials showcasing the effect of Tolvaptan in treatment of heart failure are lacking clinical findings in reduction of mortality, quality of life and re-hospitalization; other studies have evaluated its role as an adjuvant therapy in patients with volume overload and hyponatremia. An independent study in Japan showed favorable results, including increased diuresis, using Tolvaptan in patients with congestive heart failure in patients unresponsive to loop diuretics without electrolyte abnormalities within 7 days of therapy [111]. Another single center trial validated the role of Tolvaptan in the treatment of acute decompensated heart failure in addition to loop diuretics; in preventing renal injury, decreasing the required doses of diuretics and reducing the time to achieve euvolemia [112]. The AVCMA trial which studied the role of Tolvaptan vs. Carperitide (An intravenous natriuretic peptide), showed favorable results in maintaining electrolyte balance in conjunction with loop diuretics without significant hypernatremia or hemodynamic derangement [113].

The efficacy of Tolvaptan in patients with hyponatremia is well defined. Hyponatremia has been evaluated as an independent risk factor attributed to poor outcomes in patients admitted for decompensated heart failure [114]. In an era where the mainstay therapy for acute decompensated heart failure are loop diuretics; of which the most profound side effect is electrolyte abnormalities, Tolvaptan may offer a novel strategy to alleviate hyponatremia while assisting in diuresis. As mentioned before, several studies have shown the benefit of Tolvaptan in addition to loop diuretics. These studies are performed in Japan and as such cannot necessarily be generalized to other patient populations without further studies. FDA has approved the use of Tolvaptan for durations less than 30 days with recommendations against use in patients with hepatic insufficiency. It is mandated that Tolvaptan be initiated and or restarted in an inpatient setting where serum electrolytes can be monitored closely as rapid reversal of sodium concentrations can precipitate osmotic demyelination, leading to seizures, coma and death.

It is available in 15, 30 and 60 mg dosing. The recommended initial dose is 15 mg daily with titration to 30 mg after 24 h and subsequently 60 mg daily as needed to reach appropriate levels of sodium concentration. Tolvaptan is contraindicated in patients who are anuric, need an urgent rise in serum sodium, in those unable to respond to thirst, hypovolemic hyponatremia and in patients with concomitant use of strong CYP 3A inhibitors. The most common side effect of Tolvaptan noted in all clinical trials included thirst, dry mouth and polyuria. It is generally well tolerated with no significant increase in adverse effects on renal function. There are currently no guidelines for the treatment of heart failure with Tolvaptan; as such its use has been dependently driven on the comfort level of individual providers. Its efficacy in conjunction with loop diuretics, duration of therapy and the appropriate dosing remain understudied in larger patient populations within the United States. Given its relative safety profile; it is imperative for randomized clinical trials to evaluate the role of Tolvaptan from an inpatient perspective in patients with heart failure to further evaluate its efficacy in reducing symptoms, length of hospitalization, electrolyte abnormalities, renal and hepatic dysfunction and all cause mortality as an adjuvant therapy.

References

1. Go AS, Moazffarian D, Roger VL, et al. Heart disease and stroke statistics – 2013 update: a report from the American Heart Association. Circulation. 2013;127:e6–245.
2. Roger VL, Weston SA, Redfield MM, et al. Trends in heart failure incidence and survival in a community based population. JAMA. 2004;292:344–50.
3. Krumholz HM, Merrill AR, Schome EM, et al. Patterns of hospital performance in acute myocardial infarction and heart failure 30-day mortality and readmission. Circ Cardiovasc Qual Outcomes. 2009;2:407–13.
4. 2013 ACCF/AHA guideline for the management of heart failure. A report of the American College of Cardiology Foundation/

American Heart Association Task Force on Practice Guidelines. Circulation. 2013;128:e240–327.

5. Alraies MC, Tran B, Adatya S. Inotropes are linked to increased mortality in heart failure. VAD J. 1. 2015. doi:http://dx.doi.org/10.130023/VAD.2015.08.

6. Wiemer G, Scholkens BA, Becker RH, et al. Ramiprilat enhances endothelial autacoid formation by inhibiting breakdown of endothelium- derived bradykinin. Hypertension. 1991; 18:558–63.

7. The CONSENSUS Trial Study Group. Effects of enalapril on mortality in severe congestive heart failure. Results of the Cooperative North Scandinavian Enalapril Survival Study (CONSENSUS). N Engl J Med. 1987;316:1429–35.

8. Margulies KB, Barclay PL, Burnett Jr JC. The role of neutral endopeptidase in dogs with evolving congestive heart failure. Circulation. 1995;91:2036–42.

9. Ferro CJ, Spratt JC, Haynes WG, Webb DJ. Inhibition of neutral endopeptidase causes vasoconstriction of human resistance vessels in vivo. Circulation. 1998;97:2323–30.

10. Trippodo NC, Robl JA, Asaad MM, Fox M, Panchal BC, Schaeffer TR. Effects of omapatrilat in low, normal, and high renin experimental hypertension. Am J Hypertens. 1998;11(3 Pt 1):363.

11. Bevan EG, Connell JM, Doyle J, Carmichael HA, Davies DL, Lorimer AR, McInnes GT. Candoxatril, a neutral endopeptidase inhibitor: efficacy and tolerability in essential hypertension. J Hypertens. 1992;10:607–13.

12. Trippodo NC, Fox M, Monticello TM, et al. Vasopeptidase inhibition with omapatrilat improves cardiac geometry and survival in cardiomyo-pathic hamsters more than does ACE inhibition with captopril. J Cardiovasc Pharmacol. 1999;34:782–90.

13. McDowell G, Nicholls DP. The endopeptidase inhibitor, candoxatril, and its therapeutic potential in the treatment of chronic cardiac failure in man. Expert Opin Investig Drugs. 1999; 8:79–84.

14. Kostis JB, Packer M, Schmieder R, Henry D, Levy E. Omapatrilat and enalapril in patients with hypertension: the Omapatrilat Cardiovascular Treatment vs. Enalapril (OCTAVE) trial. Am J Hyperten. 2004;17:103–11.

15. Asmar R, Fredebohm W, Senftleber I, et al. Omapatrilat compared with lisinopril in treatment of hypertension as assessed by ambulatory blood pressure monitoring. J Hypertens. 2000; 18:S95.

16. Norton GR, Woodiwiss AJ, Hartford C, Trifunovic B, Middlemost S, Lee A, Allen MJ. Sustained antihypertensive actions of a dual angiotensin-converting enzyme neutral endopeptidase inhibitor, sampatrilat, in black hypertensive subjects. Am J Hypertens. 1999;12(6):563.

17. Packer M, Califf RM, Konstam MA, Krum H, McMurray JJ, Rouleau J-L, Swedberg K. Comparison of omapatrilat and enalapril in patients with chronic heart failure. The omapatrilat versus enalapril randomized trial of utility in reducing events (OVERTURE). Circulation. 2002;106:920–6.

18. Rouleau JL, Pfeffer MA, Stewart DJ, et al. Comparison of vaso-peptidase inhibitor, omapatrilat, and lisinopril on exercise toler-ance and morbidity in patients with heart failure: IMPRESS randomised trial. Lancet. 2000;356:615–20.

19. Molinaro G, Carmona AK, Juliano MA, Juliano L, Malitskaya E, Yessine MA, Chagnon M, Lepage Y, Simmons WH, Boileau G, Adam A. Human recombinant membrane-bound aminopepti-dase P: production of a soluble form and characterization using novel, internally quenched fluorescent substrates. Biochem J. 2005;385(Pt 2):389.

20. McMurray JJV, Packer M, Desai AS, Gong J, Lefkowitz MP, et al; for the PARADIGM-HF Investigators and Committees. Angiotensin-neprilysin inhibition versus enalapril in heart fail-ure. N Engl J Med. 2014;371:993–1004.

21. Gottlieb SS, Stebbins A, Voors AA, et al. Effects of neseritide and predictors of urine output in acute decompensated heart failure: results from the ASCEND-HF (acute study of clinical effectiveness of neseritide and decompensated heart failure). J Am Coll Cardiol. 2013;62:1177–83.

22. Sackner-Bernstein JD, Kowalski M, Fox M, Aaronson K. Short-term risk of death after treatment with nesiritide for decompen-sated heart failure: pooled analysis of randomized controlled trials. JAMA. 2005;293:1900–5.

23. Koller KJ, Goeddel DV. Molecular biology if the natriuretic pep-tides and their receptors. Circulation. 1992;86:1081–8.

24. Suttner S, Boldt J. Natriuretic peptide system: physiology and clinical utility. Curr Opin Crit Care. 2004;10:336–41.

25. Bestle MH, Olsen NV, Christensen P, Jensen BV, Bie P. Cardiovascular, endocrine and renal effects of urodilantin in normal humans. Am J Physiol. 1999;276(45):R684–95.

26. Marin-Grez M, Fleming JT, Steinhausen M. Atrial natriuretic peptide causes pre-glomerular vasodilation and post-glomerular vasoconstriction in rat kidney. Nature. 1986;324:473–5.

27. Baughman KL. B-type natriuretic peptide – a window to the heart. N Engl J Med. 2002;347:158–9; Stein BC, Levin RI. Natriuretic peptides: physiology, therapeutic potential and risk stratification in ischemic heart disease. Am Heart J. 1998; 135:14–23.

28. Levin ER, Gardner DG, Smason WK. Natriuretic peptides. N Engl J Med. 1998;339:321–8.

29. George M, Rajaram M, Shanmugam E, VijayaKumar TM. Novel drug targets in clinical development for heart failure. Eur J Clin Pharmacol. 2014;70:765–74.

30. deGoma EM, Vagelos RH, Fowler MB, Ashley EA. Emerging therapies for the management of decompensated heart failure. J Am Coll Cardiol. 2006;48:2397–409.

31. Hata N, et al. Effects of carperitide on the long-term prognosis of patients with acute decompensated chronic heart failure – the PROTECT multicenter randomized controlled study. Circ J. 2008;72:1787–93.

32. Mizutami T, et al. Comparison of nitrite compounds and carperitide for initial treatment of acute decompensated heart failure. Int Heart J. 2011;52:114–8.

33. Hattori H, et al. Differences in hemodynamic responses between intravenous carperitide and nicorandil in patients with acute decompensated heart failure syndromes. Heart Vessels. 2013;28:345–51.

34. Nomura F, et al. Multicenter prospective investigation on efficacy and safety of carperitide as a first-line drug for acute heart failure syndrome with preserved blood pressure – COMPASS. Circ J. 2008;72:1777–86.

35. Suwa M, et al. Mutlicenter prospective investigation on efficacy and safety of carperitide for acute heart failure in the 'real world' of therapy. Circ J. 2005;69:283–90.

36. Shculz-Knappe P, et al. Isolation and structural analysis of "urodilatin", a new peptide of the cardiodilantin-(ANP)-family, extracted from human urine. Kilm Wochenschr. 1988;66:752–9.

37. Kentsch M, et al. Hemodynamic and renal effects of urodilatin bolus injections in patients with congestive heart failure. Eur J Clin Invest. 1992;22(10):662–9.

38. Elsner D, et al. Efficacy of prolonged infusion of urodilantin [ANP-(95-126)] in patients with congestive heart failure. Am Heart J. 1995;129:766–73.

39. Mitrovic V, et al. Effects of the renal natriuretic peptide urodilantin (ularitide) in patients with decompensated chronic heart

failure: a double-blind, placebo-controlled, ascending-dose trial. Am Heart J. 2005;150:1239e.1–8.

40. Mitrovic V, et al. Hemodynamic and clinical effects of ularitide in decomensated heart failure. Eur Heart J. 2006;27: 2823–23832.

41. Luss H, et al. Renal effects of ularitide in patients with decompensated heart failure. Am Heart J. 2008;155:1012.e1–8.

42. Fevold HL, Hisaw FL, Meyer RK. The relaxative hormone of the corpus luteum. Its purification and concentration. J Am Chem Soc. 1930;106(3):3340–8.

43. Eyabalan A, Shroff SG, Novak J, et al. The vascular actions of relaxin. Adv Exp Med Biol. 2007;612:65–87.

44. Teichman SL. Relaxin, a pleiotropic vasodilator for the treatment of heart failure. Heart Fail Rev. 2009;14:321–9.

45. Teichman SL. Relaxin: review of biology and potential role in treating heart failure. Cur Heart Fail Rep. 2010;7:75–82.

46. Hsu SY, Nakabayashi K, et al. Activation of orphan receptors by the hormone relaxin. Science. 2002;295:671–4.

47. Dschietzig T, Barsch C, Richter C, et al. Relaxin, a pregnancy hormone, is a functional endothelin-1 antagonist. Circ Res. 2003;92:32–40.

48. Matthews JE, Rubin JP, Noval J, et al. Relaxin (Rix) induces fast relaxation in some rat and human arteries mediated by P13 kinase and nitric oxide. Reprod Sci. 2007;14(1 Suppl):114A.

49. Metra M, Teerlink JR, Felker GM, Greenberg BH, et al. Dsypnoea and worsening heart failure in patients with acute heart failure: results from the Pre-RELAX-AHF Study. Eur J Heart Fail. 2010;12:1130–9.

50. Teerlink JR, Cotter G, Davidson BA, Felker GM, Filippatos G, et al. Serelaxin, recombinant human relaxin-2, for treatment of acute heart failure (RELAX-AHF): a randomized, placebo-controlled trial. Lancet. 2013;381:29–39.

51. Micheletti R, Palazzo F, Barassi P, et al. Istaroxime, a stimulator of sarcoplasmic reticulum calcium adenosine triphosphate isoform 2a activity, as a novel therapeutic approach to heart failure. Am J Cardiol. 2007;99(Suppl):24A–34.

52. Braunwald E. Heart failure. J Am Coll Cardiol HF. 2013;1: 1–20.

53. Aditya S, Rattan A. Istaroxime: a rising star in acute heart failure. J Pharmacol Pharmacother. 2012;3(4):353–5.

54. Belevych AE, Terentyev D, Terentyeva R, et al. The relationship between arrhythmogenesis and impaired contractility in heart

failure: role of altered ryanodine receptor function. Cardiovasc Res. 2011;90:493–502.

55. Chen Y, Escoubet B, Prunier F, et al. Constitutive cardiac over-expression of sarcoplasmic/endoplasmic reticulum Ca2+ ATPase delays myocardial failure after myocardial infarction in rats at a cost of increase acute arrhythmias. Circulation. 2004;109:1898–903.

56. El-Armouche A, Eschenhagen T. β-adrenergic stimulation and myocardial function in the failing heart. Heart Fail Rev. 2009;14:225–41.

57. Weber CR, Piacentino III V, Houser SR, Bers DM. Dynamic regulation of sodium/calcium exchange function of failing human myocardium. Circulation. 2003;108:2224–9.

58. Micheletti R, Palazzo F, Barassi P, et al. Istaroxime, a stimulator of sarcoplasmic reticulum calcium adenosine triphosphatase isoform 2a activity, as a novel therapeutic approach to heart failure. Am J Cardiol. 2007;99(Suppl):24A–34.

59. Mattera GG, Giudice PL, Loi FM, et al. Istaroxime: a new luso-inotropic agent for heart failure. Am J Cardiol. 2007;99(Suppl): 33A–40.

60. Sabbah HN, Imai M, Cowart D, et al. Hemodynamic properties of a new-generation positive luso-inotropic agent for the acute treatment of advanced heart failure. Am J Cardiol. 2007;99(Suppl):41A–6.

61. Gheorghiade M, Blair JE, Filippatos GS, Macarie C, Ruzyllo W, et al; for the HORIZON-HF Investigators. Hemodynamic, Echocardiographic, and Neurohormonal Effects of Istaroxime, a Novel Intravenous Inotropic and Lusitropic Agent A Randomized Controlled Trial in Patients Hospitalized With Heart Failure. J Am Coll Cardiol. 2008;51:2276–85.

62. Shah SJ, Blair JE, Filippatos GS, Mecarie C, et al; for the HORIZON-HF Investigators. Effects of istaroxime on diastolic stiffness in acute heart failure syndrome: results from the Hemodynamic, Echocardiographic, and Neurohormonal Effects of Istaroxime, a Novel Intravenous Inotropic and Lusitropic Agent A Randomized Controlled Trial in Patients Hospitalized With Heart Failure. Am Heart J. 2009;157:1035–41.

63. Adamson PR, Vanoli E, Mattera GC, et al. Hemodynamic effects of a new inotropic compound, PST-2744, in dogs with chronic ischemic heart failure. J Cardiovasc Pharmacol. 2003;42:169–73.

64. Colucci WS, Wright RF, Braunwald E. New positive inotropic agents in the treatment of congestive heart failure: mechanisms

of action and recent clinical developments. N Engl J Med. 1986;314:349–58.

65. Ferrick KJ, Fein SA, Ferrick AM, et al. Effect of milrinone on ventricular arrhythmias in congestive heart failure. Am J Cardiol. 1990;66:431–4.

66. Parissis JT, Rafouli-Stergiou P, Paraskevaidis I, Mebazaa A. Levosimendan: from basic science to clinical practice. Heart Fail Rev. 2009;14:265–75.

67. Antoniades C, Tousoulis D, Koumallos N, Marinou K, Stefanadis C. Levosimendan: beyond its simple inotropic effect in heart failure. Pharmacol Ther. 2007;114:184–97.

68. Sorsa T, Heikkinen S, Abbott MB, et al. Binding of levosimendan, a calcium sensitizer, to cardiac troponin C. J Biol Chem. 2001;276:9337–43.

69. Michaels AD, McKeown B, Kostal M, Vakharia KT, Jordan MV, et al. Effects of intravenous levosimendan on human coronary vasomotor regulation, left ventricular wall stress and myocardial oxygen uptake. Circulation. 2005;111:1504–9.

70. Givertz MM, Andreou C, Conrad CH, Colucci WS. Direct myocardial effects of levosimendan in humans with left ventricular dysfunction: alteration of force-frequency and relaxation-frequency relationships. Circulation. 2007;115:1218–24.

71. Yokoshiki H, Katsube Y, Sunagawa M, et al. Levosimendan, a novel Ca 2 sensitizer, activates the glibenclamide-sensitive K-channel in rat arterial myocytes. Eur J Pharmacol. 1997;333:249–59.

72. Kivikko M, Antila S, Eha J, Lehtonen L, Pentikäinen PJ. Pharmacokinetics of levosimendan and its metabolites during and after a 24-hour continuous infusion in patients with severe heart failure. Int J Clin Pharm Ther. 2002;40:465–71.

73. Illeberg J, Laine M, Palkama T, Kivikko M, Pohjanjousi P, Kupari M. Duration of the haemodynamic action of a 24-h infusion of levosimendan in patients with congestive heart failure. Eur J Heart Fail. 2007;9:75–82.

74. Nieminen MS, Akkila J, Hasenfuss G, et al. Hemodynamic and neurohumoral effects of continuous infusion of levosimendan in patients with congestive heart failure. J Am Coll Cardiol. 2000;36:1903–12.

75. Slawsky MT, Colucci WS, Gottlieb SS, et al; for the Study Investigators. Acute hemodynamic and clinical effects of levosimendan in patients with severe heart failure. Circulation. 2000;102:2222–7.

76. Follath F, Cleland JG, Just H, et al. Efficacy and safety of intra-venous levosimendan compared with dobutamine in severe low-output heart failure (the LIDO study): a randomised double-blind trial. Lancet. 2002;360:196–202.

77. Zairis MN, Apostolatos C, Anastassiadis F, et al. Comparison of the effect of levosi-mendan,or dobutamine or placebo in chronic low output decompensated heart failure. CAlcium Sensitizer or Inotrope or NOne in low output heart failure (CASINO) study. Program and abstracts of the European Society of Cardiology, Heart Failure Update; 2004; 12–15 June; Wroclaw; 2004.

78. Mebazaa A. The Survival of patients with acute heart failure in need of IntraVEnous Inotropic Support (SURVIVE) trial. Late-breaking Clinical Trials. American Heart Association, Annual Scientific Session. Dallas; 13–16 Nov 2005.

79. Packer M. REVIVE II: multicenter placebo-controlled trial of levosimendan on clinical status in acutely decompensated heart failure. Program and abstracts from the American Heart Association Scientific Sessions 2005; 13–16 Nov 2005; Dallas: Late Breaking Clinical Trials II.

80. Urani F, Aurisicchio P, D'Ercole P. Hemodynamic and volumet-ric response to levosimendan in critical care patients. (abstract). Crit Care. 2004;6:84.

81. Delle Karth G, Buberl A, Geppert A, Neunteufl T, Huelsmann M, Kopp C, Nikfardjam M, Berger R, Heinz G. Haemodynamic effects of a continuous infusion of levosimendan in critically ill patients with cardiogenic shock requiring catecholamines. Acta Anaesthesiol Scand. 2003;47:1251–6.

82. Moiseyev VS, Poder P, Andrejevs N, Ruda MY, Golikov AP, Lazebnik LB, Kobalava ZD, Lehtonen LA, Laine T, Nieminen MS, Lie KI. RUSSLAN Study Investigators. Safety and efficacy of a novel calcium sensitizer, levosimendan, in patients with left ventricular failure due to an acute myocardial infarction. A randomized, placebo-controlled, double blind study (RUSSLAN). Eur Heart J. 2002;23:1422–32.

83. Figgitt DP, Gillies PS, Goa KL. Levosimendan. Drugs. 2001; 61(5):613–27.

84. Solaro RJ, de Tombe PP. Review focus series: sarcomeric pro-teins as key elements in integrated control of cardiac function. Cardiovasc Res. 2008;77:616–8.

85. Spudich JA. How molecular motors work. Nature. 1994;372:515–8.

86. Cohn JN, Goldstein SO, Greenberg BH, Lorell BH, Bourge RC, Jaski BE, Gottlieb SO, McGrew 3rd F, DeMets DL, White BG. A dose-dependent increase in mortality with vesnarinone

among patients with severe heart failure. Vesnarinone trial investigators. N Engl J Med. 1998;339:1810–6. doi:10.1056/NEJM199812173392503.

87. Teerlink JR. A novel approach to improve cardiac performance: cardiac myosin activators. Heart Fail Rev. 2009;14(4):289–98.

88. Malik F, Teerlink J, Escandon R, Clake C, Wolff A. The selective cardiac myosin activator, CK-1827452, a calcium-independent inotrope, increases left ventricular systolic function by increasing ejection time rather than the velocity of contraction. Circulation. 2006;114(18 Suppl):441.

89. Anderson RL, Sueoka SH, Rodriguez HM, Lee KH, Cox DR, Kawas R, Morgan BP, Sakowicz R, Morgans DJ, Malik F, Elias KA. In vitro and in vivo efficacy of the cardiac myosin activator CK-1827452. Mol Bio Cell. 2005;16.

90. Anderson RL, Pokrovskii M, Elias KA. Effects of cardiac myosin activators on excitation-contraction (E-C) coupling in ventricular myocytes. Biophysical society meeting abstracts. Biophys J. 2007;2007:133a.

91. Shen YT, Zhang Y, Morgans DJ, Vatner SF, Malik F. A novel inotropic agent that activates cardiac myosin and increases cardiac contractility without increasing MVO2 in heart failure with left ventricular hypertrophy. J Am Coll Cardiol. 2008;51(10, Suppl 1):A54. doi:10.1016/j.jacc.2008.02.004.

92. Teerlink JR, Malik FI, Clarke CP, Saikali KG, Escandon RD, Lee JH, Wolff AA. The selective cardiac myosin activator, CK-1827452, increases left ventricular systolic function by increasing ejection time: results of a first-in-human study of a unique and novel mechanism. J Card Fail. 2006;12:763.

93. Cleland JG, et al. The effects of the cardiac myosin activator, omecamtiv mecarbil, on cardiac function in systolic heart failure: a double-blind, placebo-controlled, crossover, dose-ranging phase 2 trial. Lancet. 2011;378(9792):676–83.

94. Barry HG, Will C, Rafael E, Jacqueline HL et al. Phase II Safety Study Evaluating the Novel Cardiac Myosin Activator, CK-1827452, in Patients with Ischemic Cardiomyopathy and Angina. J Card Fail. 2009;15(6). Supplement, S67.

95. Teerlink JR, Felker GM, McMurray JJV et al. Acute Treatment With Omecamtiv Mecarbil to Increase Contractility in Acute Heart Failure. The ATOMIC-AHF Study. J Am Coll Cardiol. 2016;67(12):1444–55

96. Zimmerman EA, Nilaver G, Hou-Yu A, Silverman AJ. Vasopressinergic and oxytocinergic pathways in the central nervous system. Fed Proc. 1984;43(1):91.

97. Guyton AC. The body fluids and kidneys. In: Guyton AC, Hall JE, editors. Textbook of medical physiology. Philadelphia: WB Saunders Company; 2006. p. 291–414.

98. Wade CE, Keil LC, Ramsay DJ. Role of volume and osmolality in the control of plasma vasopressin in dehydrated dogs. Neuroendocrinology. 1983;37:349–53.

99. Nielsen S, Kwon TH, Christensen BM, Promeneur D, Frøkiaer J, Marples D. Physiology and pathophysiology of renal aquaporins. J Am Soc Nephrol. 1999;10(3):647.

100. Sugimoto T, Saito M, Mochizuki S, Watanabe Y, Hashimoto S, Kawashima H. Molecular cloning and functional expression of a cDNA encoding the human V1b vasopressin receptor. J Biol Chem. 1994;269(43):27088.

101. Hibonnier M, Conarty DM, Preston JA, et al. Molecular pharmacology of human vasopressin receptors. Adv Exp Med Biol. 1998;449:251–76.

102. Yamamura Y, Nakamura S, Itoh S, et al. OPC-41061, a highly potent human vasopressin V2-receptor antagonist: pharmacological profile and aquaretic effect by single and multiple oral dosing in rats. J Pharmacol Exp Ther. 1998;287(3):860–7.

103. Rouleau JL, Packer M, Moye L, et al. Prognostic value of neurohumoral activation in patients with an acute myocardial infarction: effect of captopril. J Am Coll Cardiol. 1994;24(3):583–91.

104. Hauptman P, Zimmer C, Udelson J, et al. Comparison of two doses and dosing regimens of tolvaptan in congestive heart failure. J Cardiovasc Pharmacol. 2005;46(5):609–14.

105. Schrier RW, Gross P, Gheorghiade M, et al. Tolvaptan, a selective oral vasopressin V2 receptor antagonist, for hyponatremia. N Engl J Med. 2006;355:2099–112.

106. Gheorghiade M, Niazi I, Ouyang J, Czerwiec F, Kambayashi J, Zampino M, Orlandi C, Tolvaptan Investigators. Vasopressin V2-receptor blockade with tolvaptan in patients with chronic heart failure: results from a double-blind, randomized trial. Circulation. 2003;107(21):2690–6.

107. Gheorghiade M, Gattis WA, O'Connor C, et al. Effects of tolvaptan, a vasopressin antagonist, in patients hospitalized with worsening heart failure: a randomized controlled trial. JAMA. 2004;291:1963–71.

108. Gheorghiade M, Konstam MA, Burnett JC, et al. Short-term clinical effects of tolvaptan, an oral vasopressin antagonist, in patients hospitalized for heart failure, the EVEREST clinical status trials. JAMA. 2007;297:1332–43.

109. Udelson JE, Orlandi C, Ouyang J, Krasa H, Zimmer CA, Frivold G, Haught WH, Meymandi S, Macarie C, Raef D, Wedge P, Konstam MA, Gheorghiade M. Acute hemodynamic effects of tolvaptan, a vasopressin V2 receptor blocker, in patients with symptomatic heart failure and systolic dysfunction: an international, multicenter, randomized, placebo-controlled trial. J Am Coll Cardiol. 2008;52(19):1540–5.

110. Udelson JE, McGrew FA, Flores E, Ibrahim H, Katz S, Koshkarian G, O'Brien T, Kronenberg MW, Zimmer C, Orlandi C, Konstam MA. Multicenter, randomized, double-blind, placebo-controlled study on the effect of oral tolvaptan on left ventricular dilation and function in patients with heart failure and systolic dysfunction. J Am Coll Cardiol. 2007;49(22):2151–9.

111. Kinugawa K, Sato N, Inomata T, Shimakawa T, Iwatake N, Mizuguchi K. Efficacy and safety of tolvaptan in heart failure patients with volume overload. Circ J. 2014;78(4):844–52.

112. Shirakabe A, Hata N, Yamamoto M, Kobayashi N, Shinada T, Tomita K, Tsurumi M, Matsushita M, Okazaki H, Yamamoto Y, Yokoyama S, Asai K, Shimizu W. Immediate administration of tolvaptan prevents the exacerbation of acute kidney injury and improves the mid-term prognosis of patients with severely decompensated acute heart failure. Circ J. 2014;78(4):911–21.

113. Suzuki S, et al. Acute heart failure volume control multicenter randomized (AVCMA) trial: comparison of tolvaptan and carperitide. J Clin Pharmacol. 2013;53(12):1277–85.

114. Gheorghiade M, Abraham WT, Albert NM, et al; OPTIMIZE-HF Investigators and Coordinators. Relationship between admission serum sodium concentration, clinical outcomes in patients hospitalized for heart failure: an analysis from the OPTIMIZE-HF registry. Eur Heart J. 2007;28:980–8.

Chapter 3
A Comprehensive Transition of Care Plan for a Patient Admitted with Acute Decompensated Heart Failure

Clement C. Eiswirth

Introduction

Congestive heart failure (CHF) is a diverse syndrome (Table 3.1) encompassing multiple disease states and marked by variable rates of progression. The average hospitalized patient with heart failure (HF) faces a 1 year mortality of 30 % and a readmission rate of 50 % at 6 months [1, 2]. Acute exacerbations of chronic heart failure are common and frequently result in hospitalizations which are costly for all parties and subject hospitals to financial penalties for re-admissions. This readmission penalty is imposed regardless of the cause for the readmission and in fact, most patients are readmitted for conditions other than recurrent CHF.

C.C. Eiswirth, MD, FACC, FASE
Department of Cardiology,
Medical Director, Cardiomyopathy and Heart Failure Program,
Section of Cardiomyopathy and Heart Transplantation,
Ochsner Medical Center, Jefferson, LA, USA
e-mail: clement.eiswirth@ochsner.org

H.O. Ventura (ed.), *Pharmacologic Trends of Heart Failure*,
Current Cardiovascular Therapy,
DOI 10.1007/978-3-319-30593-6_3,
© Springer International Publishing Switzerland 2016

TABLE 3.1 Heart failure (HF) in the U.S

The leading cause of hospitalizations with one million/year

Treatment of HF costs $33 billion/year

Prevalence: five million people; 1 % in those age 50–59 years & 10 % age >75 years

Incidence 500,000 new cases/year

Stable incidence but increasing prevalence, factors include:

Aging of the population

Improved survival of cardiovascular conditions predisposing to HF

Improved survival of patients treated for HF

Earlier recognition of HF

Subsequent lifetime risk for HF for a 40 years male is 21 % & female 20 %

71 % of MI survivors over 65 years develop HF after infarct hospitalization

67 % of these HF cases present during the first year following MI

It is incumbent upon the physicians caring for these patients to implement guideline directed medical therapy (Tables 3.2) to improve patient morbidity and mortality. Progress in these efforts has translated into improvements in patient survival [3]. An effective, proven strategy to prevent readmissions remains elusive. However, there are some generally accepted methods that should be implemented including an early follow-up appointment in clinic and educating the patient about medications, diet, activity, and the warning signs and symptoms to report to the physician or their designee. One cannot emphasize enough the importance of a smooth transition when discharging a patient with congestive heart failure to the outpatient clinic. One needs to remain cognizant of the changes in the healthcare environment and the patient's desire to see a physician of their choosing. Patients discharged may have been cared for by Hospitalists or primary care physicians and may not have seen a cardiologist. They are often sent home with instructions

TABLE 3.2 Discharge summary elements for acute CHF admission

Date of admission and date of discharge

Age, gender and ethnicity

Duration of CHF and document any other admissions for CHF within the preceeding year

Type of CHF, systolic, diastolic or combined

Etiology (See Table 3.3?)

Social history to include alcohol intake, smoking, illicit drugs and caregiver support available

Admission and discharge: BP, HR, body weight, orthopnea and number of pillows used, level of JVD, degree of edema, heart rhythm, cardiac murmur, S3, hepatic congestion (span, hepatojugular reflux). If available included any change from baseline prior to the admission for these values.

Precipitating factors for the CHF episode (See Table 3.3)

Diagnostic test results and compare to baseline if available:

EKG, CXR, CMP (especially Na, K, Cr, LFTs), Mg, CBC, troponin, BNP/pro-NTBNP, urinalysis; include if performed the results of thyroid tests, iron stores, lipids, A1c

2D ECHO-doppler (if not performed then results of last test and whether one is planned as outpatient for follow-up)

Tests performed for ischemic heart disease and results if performed

Cardiac catheterization results if performed

List all cardiac devices whether implanted at this admission or previous

Pacemakers (single or dual chamber, bi-ventricular, implantable cardio-defibrillator, loop recorder, wireless PA pressure or fluid monitor

Medications upon discharge and especially important to not any changes made in the medications or their doses compared to before the admission

Activity and diet restrictions

Disposition plan and include upcoming labs and date anticipated, diagnostic tests to be performed and a comment on condition upon discharge and probability of readmission

to see a primary care physician and/or mid-level provider with or without an outpatient cardiology appointment. There are variations in the expertise of these providers in the evaluation and treatment of patient afflicted with CHF. In some cases those charged with assuming the care of the patient in the clinic did not care for the patient in the hospital. This is compounded when the medical record is not available, incomplete or not optimally documented. As part of the transition to home we must assure that these patients, who represent the sickest of the sick, are not lost in the system. A complete and thorough accounting of the hospital course and treatment plan must be documented (Table 3.2). In so doing we can better assure that these patients will continue their march to recovery in the out-patient arena.

The Scope of the Problem

Congestive heart failure (CHF) is a diverse syndrome encompassing multiple disease states and marked by variable rates of progression. This disease (Table 3.1) afflicts more than five million Americans and more than 600,000 new cases are diagnosed each year [3, 4]. Heart failure with reduced ejection fraction (HFrEF), defined as an ejection fraction (EF) of <40 % accounts for approximately half of these cases while heart failure with preserved ejection fraction (HFpEF) accounts for the remainder. HFpEF is more prevalent in women, irrespective of age and the elderly [5, 6]. Heart failure (HF) is not only the most common cause for hospital admission and re-admission in the Medicare age group but it adversely affects the quality of life of millions of Americans with a substantial morbidity and mortality. The 65 year age and sex adjusted survival for HF is lower than for most cancers including breast and prostate [7] though most patients seem to fear these cancers more than HF in the mistaken belief that HF is a more benign disease.

In the United States each year there are over 1.1 million hospitalizations for HF at a cost exceeding $20 billion. Only

10 % of the total HF population is afflicted with advanced Class D CHF. Despite this fact, 25 % of the total HF hospitalizations are due to readmissions [8, 9]. The average hospitalized patient with heart failure (HF) faces a 1 year mortality of 30 % and a readmission rate of 50 % at 6 months [1, 2, 10].

There are many factors contributing to the poor outcome of these patients including the severity of the heart failure syndrome and its etiology as well as co-morbid conditions such as age, coronary artery disease, obesity, hypertension, diabetes mellitus, chronic kidney disease, arrhythmias, anemia, chronic lung disease and obstructive sleep apnea. The complexity of the medical regimen required to care for these patients and need for a detailed plan of care including daily weights, the use of diuretics as needed based upon a body weight range assigned to the patient, dietary restrictions of salt and water all contribute to a patient's difficulty in following the treatment prescribed.

Heart failure may be aggravated by the failure of an individual to care for oneself and is frequently contributed to by the poor recognition or control of pre-existing medical problems. In many cases associated factors such as poor access to healthcare, poor socioeconomic status and lower educational levels are present. All of these contribute to the vicious cycle of recurrent heart failure.

Are Readmissions Truly the Fault of the Hospital or Physician?

Acute exacerbations of chronic heart failure are common and frequently result in hospitalizations that are costly for all parties and subject hospitals to financial penalties for readmissions. This readmission penalty is imposed regardless of the cause for the readmission. In fact, most patients are readmitted for conditions other that recurrent CHF [11]. Following the implementation of guideline directed medical therapy (GDMT) improvements in patient's morbidity and mortality are realized and in fact, progress in these efforts has translated into improvements in patient survival, symptoms and functional class [12].

Unfortunately, unadjusted, all cause readmission rates have risen from 17 % in 1993 to 20 % in 2005 [12]. Discordance between mortality and rehospitalization rates was note in the Veterans Affairs Health Care System between 2002 and 2006 [13]. In that time frame the authors noted an increase in co-morbid conditions but a stable rate of hospital admissions for HF at 5 per 1000. They observed a reduction of the in-hospital mortality rate from 4.7 to 2.8 % (p < 0.0001), a reduction in 30 day mortality from 7.1 to 5.0 % (p < 0.0001) and a reduction in 1 year mortality from 27.7 to 24.3 % (p < 0.0001). Despite these positive results, the 30 day risk for readmission rose 21 % from 2002 to 2006. These facts, have been confirmed by other studies and should give pause to those advocating all cause readmission for heart failure as a measure of quality. The results of these studies have clearly cast doubt on such a conclusion.

Steps That May Lessen Re-admission

While an effective, proven strategy to prevent readmissions remains elusive at this point, there are some generally accepted methods that should be implemented. These include an early follow-up clinic appointment (within 3–7 days) and educating the patient and caregivers. Education should thoroughly cover medications, diet and activity as well as the warning signs and symptoms that should be reported to the physician or their designee.

One of the most important measures one can perform in the care of a patient with CHF is a succinct but informative discharge summary (Table 3.2). This summary should include the age, gender and ethnicity of the patient. It is important to note how long the patient has suffered with CHF and any admissions during the preceding year for CHF. The etiology of the heart failure should be identified, e.g. ischemia, valvular, non-ischemic, etc. as well as the mechanism of HF (systolic, diastolic or both). Pertinent social history such as

TABLE 3.3 Conditions that can precipitate acute decompensated HF

Coronary artery disease with ischemia and/or infarction

Atrial fibrillation, flutter, ventricular tachycardia, bradycardia with or without AV block, etc)

Uncontrolled hypertension

Anemia

Infection

Exacerbation of chronic lung disease with or without pneumonia

Pulmonary embolism

Adverse effects of medications (NSAIDs, calcium channel blockers, prednisone, TZDs, etc.)

Non-compliance with medications and/or diet

Thyroid disorder

Anemia

Substance abuse

smoking, alcohol, illicit drug use as well as employment factors and caregiver support should be included.

Identified precipitating factors (Table 3.3) for the patient's hospitalization with ADHF should be included in the summary. The admission and discharge blood pressure, pulse and body weight should be recorded. The presence of orthopnea and the number of pillows required for comfortable breathing is documented in the summary as well the level of jugular vein distension (JVD), the grade of peripheral edema and evidence of hepatic congestion. This should include a determination of the liver size (finger-breadths below right costal margin or the span by percussion) and the presence or absence of hepato-jugular reflux. One should next document the presence or absence of a heart murmur and/or S3. It is prudent to record any changes in the admission exam compared to these findings prior to admission (if known) as well as those physical exam findings noted at the time of discharge.

The results of all diagnostic tests such as EKG, CXR, ECHO, stress testing, catheterization results, etc. should be listed and compared to prior studies. The admission and discharge labs should be listed for comparison as this will also assist in follow-up care. A list of any cardiac devices present before or inserted during the admission should be supplied in the summary. Most importantly, a detailed list of medications to include the strength of the pill and the prescribed dose along with any changes in medications or dosing from prior to admit should be documented. Activity, diet and disposition need to be included along with any diagnostic testing planned for after the discharge. A thorough discharge summary will help the physician responsible for the care of the patient in their assumption of care and assure a smooth transition in the outpatient arena.

Heart Failure Disease Management

In an effort to improve the morbidity and mortality associated with HF and reduce readmission rates, heart failure disease management (HFDM) programs have been developed and introduced to hospitals across the country. These programs are designed to improve the implementation of and compliance with guideline directed medical therapy (GDMT). The successful program works with patients to improve their compliance with medications, diet and activity by identifying barriers and addressing these with the patient and/or caregivers. Through education one should increase the skills of the patient and his caregiver for self directed management. These efforts coupled with providing easy access to providers around the clock should reduce the utilization rate of the emergency department or hospital and reduce the cost of care.

While the results of individual studies of HFDM have been mixed, published meta-analyses [14, 15] have demonstrated a 20–30 % reduction in hospital readmission rates at 3–6 months and a 20 % improvement in survival. This is associated with improved medication adherence, improvements in quality of life and a reduction in the cost of care. While all patients with

HF should be approached with these general principles, the patients most likely to benefit from a HFDM program would be those at higher risk of morbidity, mortality or readmission. These would include those patients at discharge with persistent congestion, NYHA Class III or IV symptoms, those who have experienced 2 hospitalizations in 6 months or 3 in 1 year, history of prior non-compliance with diet restrictions, medications and/or daily weights. Other risk factors include depression, cognitive impairment or the presence of multiple co-morbidities especially chronic kidney (disease stage 3 or more), diabetes mellitus and chronic pulmonary disease [16].

A typical HFDM program is composed of cardiologists, mid-levels or registered nurses with specialized HF training. It is imperative that the HFDM program have easy access to social workers, dieticians, home health services, financial counselors, physical and occupational therapists and pharmacists. This group is responsible for providing each patient with a tailored medical program that optimizes GDMT. This program must include instructions for the patient to follow regarding management of dehydration (nausea, vomiting and/or diarrhea), congestion (worsening dyspnea, edema and/or orthopnea) or changes in body weight. This program will provide the patient with around the clock support, patient education, an updated list of medications and the purpose of each medication as well as make suggestions on ways to improve compliance. Some helpful actions include the use of patient logs documenting changes in body weight, symptoms and diuretic dosing adjustments as a result, pill dispensers, and prescribing home health care if necessary.

How Can We Target the Development of Heart Failure?

The most common cause for both admission and readmission of the heart failure patient is congestion. Therefore, the relief of congestion is the most important factor to target to achieve patient comfort and lessen the risk of re-admission to the hospital [4, 17–19]. It is intuitive that one should maximize the mobilization of fluid and relieve congestion in the hospitalized patient and assure the maintenance of this success in the outpatient arena.

One of the most critical challenges facing physicians treating patients afflicted with HF is whether one can successfully predict the occurrence of or detect the onset of decompensated HF. If one identifies a group of patients at high risk for developing decompensated heart failure that model should also help predict those at risk for recurrent hospitalization. Once these patients are identified then a specific program to serve them should be implemented. A successful program will improve the patient's quality of life and prevent readmissions.

If one could identify the onset of ADHF before the onset of symptoms and implement a timely change in therapies that should improve the patient's condition such that hospitalization can be avoided. A successful intervention may also improve patient outcomes beyond hospitalization rates since one knows that decompensated HF resulting in a first or repeat hospitalization portends a worse prognosis [20]. While one could argue an observational bias that the sickest patients are the ones hospitalized and hence that is the reason for the worse prognosis, troponin release associated with decompensated heart failure may better explain this finding.

Clinically it has long been speculated that daily weights would assist the patient and the clinician in identifying the onset of acute decompensated heart failure. Unfortunately, that has not been uniformly helpful in identifying and managing these patients. The author does not use the recommendation that patients call for a 3 pound weight gain overnight or 5 pounds in a week. Too many patients given this instruction develop decompensated heart failure and present to the clinic, emergency department or hospital after gaining more than 10 pounds. They do not call as the weight is gained slowly such that by following these instructions literally the threshold to call is not reached. Instead, assigning the patient a target dry weight with instructions in the use of a sliding scale diuretic regimen is critical for successful management.

Patients should be instructed to weigh each morning upon arising from sleep after voiding and prior to the oral intake of medications, food or liquids. The weight should be obtained while in underwear, light night clothing or naked. If they gain 3 or more pounds from their assigned dry weight then a self-directed increase in oral diuretics and if appropriate potassium supplementation should be implemented that morning. If they fail to respond to this measure or gain more than 5 pounds over the assigned dry weight then a more aggressive diuretic regimen should be undertaken. At that point one might consider a further increase in the dose of the loop diuretic, changing to a different loop diuretic (Table 3.6), adding a thiazide diuretic or arranging for the administration of a parenteral loop diuretic. The latter could be accomplished with an intramuscular or intravenous route of administration in the home or clinic.

Effectively Treating Congestive Heart Failure, a Brief Overview for the Transition Phase

One can see that with over one million hospitalizations for CHF in the United States [1] and recognizing a 25–30 % rehospitalization [11] rate, even a 10 % reduction in readmissions would yield an estimated savings of $1 billion. The drug treatment of heart failure (Table 3.5) is well established but the treatment should also include the education of the patient and caregiver in this disease. Instructions in the prompt recognition of symptoms, dietary restrictions, lifestyle modifications, abstinence from or judicious use of alcohol, smoking cessation, immunization (influenza and pneumonia), activity, exercise training and maintenance of body weight is critical. In female patients, counseling regarding pregnancy in conjunction with reasonable options for birth control requires a thorough discussion.

TABLE 3.4 Drug therapy for chronic heart failure

Beta-blockers
Angiotensin converting enzyme inhibitors (ACE)
Angiotensin receptor blockers (ARB)
Neprilysin inhibitor in combination with an ARB[a]
Digoxin
Hydralazine/nitrates
Diuretics
I-f channel blockers[a]
Anti-thrombotics
Statin therapy
Anti-arrhythmics only if mandatory
Limited to two agents, amiodarone and dofetilide
Drugs to avoid
Non-steroidal anti-inflammatory drugs
Thiazolidinediones
Aspirin, unless absolutely indicated
Calcium channel blockers
Except for amlodipine if mandatory for ischemia or hypertension

[a]These agents have been recently approved in the U.S and are not currently included in national guidelines for management of CHF

The initiation of an angiotensin converting enzyme inhibitor (ACE) (Table 3.5) or angiotensin receptor blocker (ARB) (Table 3.6) in those patients whom are ACE intolerant during the index hospitalization is very important in the care of these patients. Aldosterone antagonists (Table 3.7) should be added either in the hospital or in the clinic during follow-up.

Beta blocker therapy with one of the approved agents for CHF (Table 3.8) should be implemented in the hospital setting once the patient is off intravenous diuretics and

TABLE 3.5 Recommended doses for ACE inhibitors in HF

ACE	Intial	Target
Captopril	6.25 mg TID	50 mg TID
Enalapril	2.5 mg BID	20 mg BID
Lisinopril	2.5–5 mg QD	20–40 mg QD
Benazepril	10 mg QD	80 mg QD
Ramipril	2.5 mg QD	10 mg QD
Quinapril	5 mg BID	20 mg BID
Fosinopril	5–10 mg QD	40 mg QD

TABLE 3.6 Recommended doses for ARB'S in HF

ARB	Initial	Target
Losartan	25–50 mg QD	50–100 mg QD
Losartan included in the guidelines however, the author believes that the		
Data for this drug is weaker than for the other listed ARB'S		
If used suggest target dose of 150 mg		
Valsartan	40 mg BID	160 mg BID
Do not use as add on therapy in patients already receiving a beta blocker		
With an ace due to higher mortality in this group		
Candesartan	4–8 mg QD	32 mg QD

congestion has resolved. In a patient admitted with ADHF who requires an inotrope, the beta-blocker should not be initiated until the inotrope has been discontinued. In these cases it is reasonable to delay initiating this therapy until the first clinic visit to allow time to assure that they are hemodynamically stable. The beta-blocker should be titrated to the target dose with an incremental change no sooner than 2 week intervals until a resting heart rate

TABLE 3.7 Recommended aldosterone antagonist[a] in HF

Drug	Initial	Target
Spironolactone[b]	12.5 mg QD	50 mg QD
Eplerenone[b,c]	+25 mg QD	50 mg QD

[a]Do not use if K > 5.0 or GFR <30; monitor K at 1 week, 1 month and Q3 months
[b]If patient not on ACE or ARB then consider doubling these doses
[c]Gynecomastia occurred in 10 % of patients in rales trial; eplerenone is less likely to cause this since it has a much lower affinity for the sex hormone recpetors

TABLE 3.8 Recommended doses for beta blockers in HF

Beta blocker	Initial	Target
Carvedilol	3.125 mg BID	25–50 mg BID
Metoprolol succinate	12.5–25 mg QD	200 mg QD
Bisoprolol	1.25 mg QD	10 mg QD
Nebivolol (not approved in U.S.)	1.25 mg QD	10 mg QD

below 70 bpm is achieved, the patient exhibits intolerance to a higher dose or the maximal dose of the beta-blocker has been reached.

If the patient has atrial fibrillation it is critical that rate control be established prior to discharge. The optimal target rate at rest for atrial fibrillation in heart failure has not been determined though generally accepted to be below 80 bpm. Whether patients with persistent or chronic atrial fibrillation and heart failure with reduced ejection fraction attain a benefit from the use of the beta-blockers currently approved in the U.S. is unknown. This controversy arises from the results of retrospective analyses of the trials leading to the approval of these agents [21–24]. Nonetheless, beta-blockers are recommended and used in these patients as they are the most effective agents to achieve rate control in patients with atrial fibrillation. The dose should be adjusted to target the ventricular rate to below 80 beats per minute.

Ivabradine [25], is a newly approved agent for the treatment for HFrEF and acts to selectively inhibit the If current in the sinoatrial (SA) node. Inhibition of this channel results in a slowing repolarization of the SA node and thereby slowing the heart rate. This agent has no effect on AV nodal conduction and therefore should not be prescribed in patients with atrial fibrillation or flutter as it will not slow the ventricular rate in these cases. Anticoagulation should be accomplished in patients with HF and atrial fibrillation or flutter to lessen the risk of an embolic event. An attempt to restore sinus rhythm should be made in most patients with CHF in the absence of chronic atrial fibrillation. If this is not performed during the index hospitalization then arrangements should be made as an outpatient and documented. If one elects to control the rate and maintain atrial fibrillation as the rhythm of choice in these patients then documentation supporting the rationale for this approach should be clearly stated in the medical record.

Determining the diuretic dose for home can sometimes be challenging. Higher doses are required at worse levels of renal function. Dividing the total daily dose of the intravenous loop diuretic by 3 and administering that amount twice daily can be used as a rough estimate. For instance, a patient on a furosemide infusion at 10 mg/h is receiving 240 mg/day. The expected home dose for this patient is 80 mg twice daily. If the patient was on a loop diuretic prior to admission a reasonable consideration would be to increase the daily dose by 1.5–2.0 fold initially or consider changing to an alternative loop diuretic. The patient should be observed at least 24 h on the chosen oral diuretic regimen to assure stability of volume status, renal function and electrolytes.

They should have assessment of renal function and electrolytes within 3–7 days of discharge along with an outpatient clinic visit. A simple question inquiring how dependent the patient is on the presence of restroom facilities for 4–6 h following an oral dose of a loop diuretic gives one a rough guide as to the effectiveness of the chosen dose. If the dose prescribed is not resulting in an effective dieresis it is likely that the tubular threshold has not been reached and increasing

TABLE 3.9 Commonly used diuretics for heart failure

Drug	Initial	Typical dose
Furosemide	20–40 mg per day	40–240 mg per day
Bumetanide	0.5–1.0 mg per day	1.0–5.0 mg per day
Torsemide	5–10 mg per day	10–20 mg per day
Ethacrynic acid	25–50 mg per day	200 mg per day
Metolazone	2.5 mg per day	2.5–10.0 mg per day
Chlorthalidone	12.5–25 mg per day	100–200 mg per day
Hctz	25–50 mg per day	200 mg per day
Indapamide	2.5 mg per day	5 mg per day

the dose, changing to a different loop diuretic or adding a thiazide diuretic is required. A list of commonly used diuretics and dose ranges is included in Table 3.9.

After Medical Treatment Is the Transition Complete?

A discussion of additional strategies that one might implement to accomplish the ultimate goal of improving the survival and quality of life of these patients while avoiding recurrent hospitalizations is required. The physician must remember the scope of this problem with over five million people in the United States carrying a diagnosis of CHF and over 550,000 new cases are diagnosed each year [3]. It is the most common Medicare DRG and the cost of caring for this disease exceeds $30 billion annually. Healthcare projections are that this cost will continue to rise as the prevalence of HF is expected to continue to increase as the population ages. This increased prevalence is also fueled by improvements in the survival of victims of acute myocardial infarction, more successful treatment of valvular heart disease and improved survival into adulthood of patients with complex congenital heart disease.

Work to End the Cycle of Heart Failure as Part of the Transition

Heart failure begets heart failure and hospitalizations signal a patient with a worsening prognosis especially in the face of recurrent hospitalizations. This is likely fueled by the complex interactions involving the renin-angiotensin-aldosterone system (RAAS), the sympathetic nervous system (SNS), adverse effects of an activated inflammatory state and oxidative stress as well as adverse vascular adaptations. Elevated troponin levels correlate with prognosis and likely reflect ongoing myocardial necrosis that occurs in some patients with chronic HF and those requiring admission for decompensated HF. Hypertension, myocardial infarction and diabetes mellitus contribute to 90 % of HF cases [26]. Effective treatment of hypertension, diabetes mellitus, hyperlipidemia and obesity as well as avoidance and cessation of tobacco using established national guidelines can help prevent the onset and recurrence of CHF [27].

The syndrome of HF is complex and the underlying etiology as well as the presence of aggravating conditions influences the outcome of these patients. One should document and address these conditions in the hospital and/or document a plan to address them as part of the transition from inpatient to outpatient care. It is critical that the etiology of the patient's HF (Table 3.10) be determined and documented before discharge. A search for coronary artery disease, ischemia, valvular heart disease, congestive cardiomyopathy, familial cardiomyopathy, myocarditis, arrhythmias, infiltrative or hypertrophic cardiomyopathy is critical. One should also evaluate for any aggravating conditions including anemia, arrhythmias, sleep apnea, lung disease and/or hypoxemia, infection and thyroid disorders. If they are identified effective treatment should be initiated prior to discharge and a documented plan for outpatient care must be included in the discharge summary.

TABLE 3.10 Etiologies of cardiomyopathy/CHF

Coronary artery disease/prior MI

Hypertension

Idiopathic dilated cardiomyopathy

Familial cardiomyopathy

   Hypertrophic cardiomyopathy

   Left ventricular non-compaction

   Arrhythmogenic right ventricular cardiomyopathy

   Familial dilated cardiomyopathy

Endocrine related:

   Hyopthyroidism

   Hyperthyroidism

   Diabetes mellitus

   Pheochromocytoma

Peripartal cardiomyopathy

Tachycardia induced

   Uncontrolled ventricular rate of atrial fibrillation

   Uncontrolled ventricular rate of atrial flutter

   Uncontrolled ventricular rate of atrial tahcycardia

   Frequent premature ventricular contractions

Valvular heart disease

Toxic cardiomyopathy

   Chemotherapy induced

   Alcohol induced

   Cocaine induced

TABLE 3.10 (continued)

Infectious
Chagas disease
HIV associated
Myocarditis
Amyloidosis
Familial TTR mutation
Wild type TTR
AL

EVALUATIONS THAT MUST BE ACCOMPLISHED AS AN INPATIENT OR ORDERED FOR THE TRANSITION TO OUTPATIENT CARE

In the initial evaluation it is critical that the ejection fraction be determined before formulating a long term treatment strategy. The single most important test in the evaluation of HF is an echocardiogram. Whether a patient has heart failure with preserved ejection fraction (HFpEF) or reduced ejection fraction (HFrEF) is an important clinical distinction for the implementation of GDMT though this distinction has a minimal impact on prognosis. The 1 year mortality rate with HFpEF is 22–29 % versus 30–50 %with HFrEF while the 5 year mortality rate is 65 % versus 70–80 % respectively [5]. An EKG should be performed in all patients presenting with HF to determine the cardiac rhythm, to assess for atrial or ventricular hypertrophy, to assess for evidence of ischemia or infarction, to identify any underlying conduction disturbances and to determine the QTc interval. In patients with chest pain, EKG evidence of ischemia or infarction and/or echo evidence of segmental wall motion abnormality the performance of angiography should be entertained if the patient is a suitable candidate for revascularization.

Endomyocardial biopsy should be considered in patients presenting with acute, fulminate HF of undetermined etiology of less than 2 weeks duration who continue to deteriorate despite conventional therapy. Endomyocardial biopsy is indicated in patients with HF of 2–12 weeks duration associated with left ventricular dilatation, complex ventricular arrhythmias and/or second or third degree heart block who fail to respond to standard care of HF in 2–3 weeks. Other indications include unexplained restrictive cardiomyopathy and if eosinophilic myocarditis or anthracycline cardiotoxicity is suspected [28]. Since this procedure is rarely indicated during the initial hospitalization for ADHF, it is important to remember its role in assessing these patients as the decision to perform a biopsy will likely be made in the early phase of outpatient care.

Methods to Determine the Prognosis of Patients with ADHF

The patient's prognosis should be determined prior to hospital discharge recognizing that in some this is difficult as it will require a period of time on therapy before an accurate assessment can be performed. Nonetheless, it is prudent that the physician attempt to determine the prognosis upon admission and discharge, expounding upon this as the patient is followed in the outpatient arena by observing their response to therapy. Appropriate identification of patients who would realize a functional and survival benefit from cardiac resynchronization therapy (CRT) generally with the implantation of a cardio-defibrillator is critical to the care of these patients. If they meet the indication for the device and fail to respond to medical therapy within 3 months then one should proceed with implantation. Therefore this is another critical step to document as one formulates the plan for the transitioning the patient to the outpatient clinic.

Determing the Prognosis of Patients Admitted with ADHF

Acute decompensated heart failure (ADHF) is a clinical presentation of heart failure necessitating care which is received in an unscheduled clinic visit or an urgent care or emergency room setting. In the vast majority of the cases the patient has a prior history of CHF and the others represent new onset heart failure most frequently caused by an acute coronary syndrome. Other precipitating factors can be uncontrolled hypertension, acute arrhythmias particularly atrial fibrillation, acute valvular heart disease chiefly mitral insufficiency from mitral valve prolapse with acute chordal rupture, peripartal cardiomyopathy, myocarditis and stress induced (takaotsubo) cardiomyopathy. The patient typically presents with acute congestive symptoms such as dyspnea, orthopnea and/or edema but can present with less obvious symptoms such as abdominal discomfort, fatigue and easy satiety. Over the years physicians have searched for reliable methods to determine the prognosis of patients afflicted with ADHF as well as chronic HF.

In keeping with this effort a large cohort of patients from the Acute Decompensated Heart Failure National Registry (ADHERE) [29] were reviewed to determine prognostic features. In this effort it was noted that BUN, systolic blood pressure (SBP) and serum creatinine (Cr) were all predictors of survival. The best single predictor of mortality was an elevated BUN $\geq$43 mg/dl and in these patients the 1 year mortality was 9.0 % versus 2.7 %. Further differentiation of the mortality rate was possible by adding SBP to the analysis. To interpret this data more easily it is important to note that in patients admitted with ADHF, an elevated BP portends a better prognosis for surviving the hospital stay while impaired renal function portends a worse prognosis [30]. Therefore, as expected in patients with a SBP $\geq$115 mmHg and a BUN $\geq$43 mg/dl, mortality rate fell to 6.4 %. If one had both BUN

≥43 mg/dl and SBP <115 mmHg the mortality rate increased to 15.3 %. In the subset with both high risk features of an elevated BUN and lower SBP as defined, adding serum Cr helped further define the mortality risk. In these cases if the serum Cr was <2.75 mg/dl then the observed mortality was slightly better at 12.4 %. On the other hand, the mortality jumped to 21.9 % in those with Cr ≥2.75 mg/dl. In the lower risk group of patients with BUN <43 mg/dl (mortality 2.7 %) who had the higher risk feature of SBP <115 mmHg the mortality rate rose to 5.5 % while in those whose SBP ≥115 mmHg the mortality rate was only 2.1 %. In another large trial, The Organized Program to Initiate Lifesaving Treatment in Hospitalized Patients with Heart Failure (OPTIMIZE-HF) [31] it was noted that the two most powerful predictors of in-hospital mortality were systolic BP ≤100 mmHg and serum Cr ≥2.0 mg/dl. These findings are consistent with the ADHERE analysis and support the use of routinely measured admission data of SBP and renal function to identify those at high risk for in-hospital mortality. Since the higher risk patients surviving the hospitalization would likely represent a higher risk group of outpatients, these profiles have implications for outpatient management and are important to remember during the transition of care.

Defining Congestion in Heart Failure

There are additional clinical models that attempt to quantify congestion that are important for the clinician to use in patients with HF. The EVEREST trial [32, 33] enrolled patients admitted to the hospital for worsening heart failure with reduced ejection fraction. Enrollees had NYHA Class III or IV symptoms plus two or more symptoms or signs of congestion. Congestion was defined as dyspnea, edema or the presence of jugular venous distension (JVD). Patients were seen daily and assessed for dyspnea, orthopnea, fatigue, JVD, rales and edema. Each of these was graded on a four point

scale (0–3) and a composite congestion score (CCS) was calculated by summing the scores for each finding. Dyspnea, orthopnea and fatigue were given a score of 0=none, 1=seldom,
2=frequent and 3=continuous. JVD was assessed in cm of
water and awarded 0 points for ≤6 cm, 1 point for 6–9 cm, 2
points for 10–15 cm, 3 points for ≥15 cm. A physical exam for
rales was performed and graded as 0 points=no rales, 1
point=only basal rales, 2 points=rales confined to lower half
of chest but more extensive than basal rales, 3 points=rales
extending into the upper half of the chest. The presence of
edema was graded as 0 points=absent/trace, 1 point=mild, 2
points=moderate and 3 points=marked. Patients were followed for a median of 9.9 months. Patients with a CCS at discharge of 0 versus a score of 3–9 experienced an increased rate
of hospitalizations for heart failure (HHF), 26.2 % versus
34.7 % and all cause mortality (ACM), 19.1 % versus 42.8 %.
After adjusting for potential confounders discharge CCS was
associated with an increased risk of ACM as well as ACM + HHF
at 30 days and for the study duration. The CCS was not associated with 30 day HHF but it was at completion of the study. A
discharge CCS of 0–2 points versus 3–9 points exhibited similar
reductions in body weight (2.2 kg versus 2.0 kg) but patients
with a discharge CCS of 3–9 points demonstrated higher levels
of BNP (423 versus 929) and NT-proBNP (2581 versus 4437)
at discharge. Scores at discharge of 0 correlated with the best
outcomes in terms of hospitalizations for heart failure (HHF)
26.2 %, all cause mortality (ACM) 19.1 % and the combination
of ACM + HHF 35.6 %. This contrasted sharply with outcomes
for scores of 3–9 which demonstrated rates for HHF 34.7 %,
ACM 42.8 % and ACM + HHF 60.0 % [34].

A similar evaluation known as the orthodema score was
formulated in an attempt to quantify and monitor congestion
in the hospital but should also be useful in the outpatient setting [35]. A post hoc retrospective analysis of the Insights
From Diuretic Optimization Strategy Evaluation in Acute
Decompensated Heart Failure (DOSE-AHF) and the
Cardiorenal Rescue Study in Acute Decompensated Heart

Failure (CARRESS-HF) demonstrated its value as a target for therapy. The score is calculated using only edema and orthopnea. It is easily determined by members of the health-care team, the patients and/or family members. Edema is graded as trace or mild (0 points), moderate (1 point) or severe (3 points). Orthopnea is determined by inquiring if the patient requires at least two pillows to be comfortable sleeping (yes = 2 points; no = 0 points). Scores of 0 represent no congestion, 1–2 represent low-grade congestion and 3–4 represent high grade congestion. While event rates were high for all scores due to the poor prognosis of heart failure, the higher the orthodema score the worse the outcome. The authors observed a 50 % rate of death, rehospitalization or unscheduled clinic visit with a score of 0, 52 % with score of 1–2 and 68 % with a score of 3–4, P = 0.038. The higher the orthodema score on admission the longer the length of stay, 7.1 days (score 1–2) versus 8.9 days (score 3–4), P = 0.004. Interestingly, there was no statistically significant difference observed in the weight lost by the patient during the hospital stay for an admission orthodema score of 1–2 versus 3–4. This supports the contention that there are factors other than solely fluid status contributing to the decompensated heart failure state that force the patient to seek hospital care for the relief of symptoms. These observations lend further support to targeting congestion as a treatment endpoint as its resolution portends a better survival [36, 37].

Clinical Scores Consistent with Invasively Obtained Risk Models: The Prognosis Determined Should Impact Therapeutic Decisions in the Transition to Outpatient Care

Swan Ganz catheters are not routinely inserted for the management of heart failure patients since the publication of the ESCAPE Trial [38]. Therefore it is incumbent upon the clinician to rely on other clinical and laboratory assessments to determine the risk the patient faces for mortality and morbidity over the ensuing months. The clinician must also synthesize the available information from the history, physical exam and laboratory data on hepatic and renal function to estimate cardiac filling pressures and the adequacy of systemic perfusion. This information allows the clinician to determine the best treatment options for the individual patient, i.e. diuretics and/or vasodilators with or without the initiation of an inotrope. These determinations will also help the physician responsible for transitioning the patient to home as they reflect upon the patient's prognosis. Determining this prognosis and relaying this information to the patient and the physician assuming the responsibility for the outpatient care is a critical step in the transition process.

Proportional pulse pressure (PPP) can be used as a non-invasive estimate of cardiac index (CI). It is calculated by dividing the pulse pressure (systolic BP-diastolic BP) by the systolic BP. The PPP correlates directly to the CI and lower values correlate with worsening prognosis. This relationship starts at PPP of ≤0.40 and is especially true at a value of ≤0.25 where it strongly correlates to CI ≤2.2 l/min/m^2 [39–41].

Dr. Forrester and colleagues published invasive hemodynamic subsets to guide the treatment of patients with an acute myocardial infarction in the 1970's using pulmonary capillary wedge pressure (PCWP) and cardiac index (CI) [42, 43]. In 2003 Dr. Stevenson [44] validated a clinical assessment that correlates with the Forrester hemodynamic profiles and allows one to predict patient outcomes in acute heart failure states non-invasively. This determination requires the clinician to assess for the presence or absence of both congestion and adequate perfusion. Congestion was considered present if there was a recent history of orthopnea and/or neck vein distension, rales, ascites, hepatojugular reflux, edema, leftward radiation of the pulmonic heart sound or demonstration of a square wave blood pressure response to the Valsalva maneuver. Inadequate perfusion was determined by any of the following, a PPI ≤0.25, pulsus alternans, symptomatic hypotension (excluding orthostatic hypotension), cool extremities or impaired mental status. Patients were considered to be dry and warm if there was no evidence of congestion or impaired perfusion (Profile A), wet and warm if there was congestion but normal perfusion (Profile B), dry and cold if there was no congestion but evidence for impaired perfusion (Profile L) and wet and cold if there was both congestion and impaired perfusion (Profile C). As expected, patients with Profile C had the worst survival followed by Profile B. The best survival was in Profile A. While the Kaplan Meir curve for Profile L was better than for Profiles B & C, due to small number of patients in the profile the authors were unable to conclude with certainty the significance of this finding. The survival of these groups corresponds well to those of Forrester using hemodynamic subsets to identify similar groups of acute MI patients. In his work patients were divided into four groups, warm and dry (CI >2.2, PCWP ≤18 mmHg), warm and wet (CI >2.2, PCWP >18), cool and dry (CI ≤2.2, PCWP ≤18 mmHg) and cool and wet (CI ≤2.2, PCWP >18 mmHg). These profiles correspond to Stevenson's profiles A, B, L and C respectively.

Non-invasive Risk Scores That Help in the Transition of Care by Assiting the Physician in Determining Prognosis

The Heart Failure Survival Score (HFSS) [45] was developed to assess the prognosis of patients referred for cardiac transplantation. It uses seven clinical variables to define low, medium and high risk subsets of patients. The variables are resting heart rate, mean blood pressure, the presence of QRS duration >120 ms regardless of cause, serum sodium level, presence of ischemic heart disease, left ventricular ejection fraction and peak oxygen consumption (VO2 max). The survival rates at 1 year were 93%, 72% and 43% in the low, medium and high risk groups.

The value of this model has been called into question since it was developed before the wide spread implementation of beta-blocker and device therapy in clinical practice. This group subsequently published data examining the effects of beta-blocker use on the predictive value of the HFSS [46]. As expected in this study, the patients receiving beta-blockers had better 1 and 2 year survival (90.3 and 85.6 %) compared to those not receiving beta-blockers (75.7 and 63.7 %), p <0.0001. For patients not on a beta-blocker but with a low risk HFSS score the 1 and 2 year survival rates were 88.5 and 84.5 % while those on beta blocker had survival rates at 1 and 2 years of 95.1 and 94.1 %. For the medium risk score without beta-blocker 1 and 2 year survival rates were 81.8 and 61.8 % while those on beta blocker had survival rates at 1 and 2 years of 85.8 and 78.9 %. For the high risk score without beta-blocker 1 and 2 year survival rates were 46.8 and 32.1 % while those on beta blocker had survival rates at 1 and 2 years of 83.1 and 59.8 %. The p values across all strata were highly significant, p < 0.0001. In using the HFSS it is important for the reader to note that these were ambulatory outpatients who were able to perform a cardiopulmonary stress exercise test and reach their anaerobic threshold. Interested parties can access this calculator free of charge at http://handheld.softpedia.com/get/Health/Calculator/HFSS-Calc-37354.shtml.

Another useful computer based model is the Seattle Heart Failure Prognostication Model [47, 48] developed by Levy and colleagues at the University of Washington Health Sciences Center. The model has been updated to include all GDMT options and device therapy. One can use this model to project a patient's 1, 2 and 3 year survival and the impact of various interventions on these estimates. Of course it is important to recognize the limitations of all predictive models and in the experience of this author, this model overestimates survival. Nonetheless, it is extremely useful in demonstrating the relative risk reductions an individual patient would be expected to realize if they underwent certain medical or device related therapeutic interventions. One can use this model to educate the patient and caregiver on the impact these therapies have in their case and in so doing might improve compliance with the plan of care that the physician is recommending. This model can be accessed at http://SeattleHeartFailureModel.org and the service is free of charge.

The Role of Biomarkers in the Transition of Care and in Predicting Prognosis

Biomarkers are a diverse group of biological substances that can be measured and reflect underlying pathologic or physiologic states. To be a clinically useful biomarker three general concepts must be fulfilled. First, the substance detected should be accurately and reproducibly measured in a cost-effective manner with the result readily available to the attending physician; second, it should provide the clinician with information not already available from the clinical assessment; third, the result should assist the treatment team in determining the medical care to be rendered [49]. There are a variety of biomarkers identified for patients with HF that reflect inflammation, oxidative stress, neurohormonal activation, myocyte injury, myocyte stretch and macrophage activation. A complete discussion of biomarkers is beyond the scope of this chapter but interested parties might review Dr. Braunwald's paper, Biomarkers in Heart Failure published in 2008 [50].

The natriuretic peptides generally available in practice are B-type natriuretic peptide (BNP) and N-terminal pro-BNP (NT-proBNP) levels. There is no debate that if the diagnosis of CHF is in doubt measuring one of these markers can improve the diagnostic certainty of CHF or alternatively assist the clinician in excluding its presence [51, 52]. The release of these compounds depends upon wall stress and mechanical stretch thus levels for HFpEF are lower than with HFrEF. The absolute levels are associated with the prognosis in patients with

HFrEF. Interpretation of these levels requires a knowledge of conditions and factors that can impact the result. The levels of these markers can be increased by acute or chronic kidney disease, myocardial infarction, pulmonary embolism, cor pulmonale and electrical cardioversion. The levels are also higher in females than males and increase with advancing age. These levels can be artificially low in overweight patients. Also, since their release depends upon wall stress the observed values are lower in HFpEF than HFrEF patients.

Using these markers to guide therapy has yielded mixed results and the outcome changes noted are due to the attainment of GDMT. In two meta-analyses of randomized controlled trials using biomarker guided therapy, an increase in the prescribed doses for ACE/ARB, aldosterone antagonists and beta-blockers was seen when physicians had access to BNP and NT-proBNP levels. Interestingly, in the six trials reviewed there was no significant increase in diuretic dosages employed in response to these biomarkers. Also, the changes in the drug therapies mentioned above did not result in an increase in adverse events including hypotension or renal impairment. The patients in the control group were also well treated with similar percentages of patients prescribed these agents though presumably not on target doses. There was no explanation for the failure to prescribe target doses in these patients. There was a 31 % improvement in mortality in the meta-analysis in the arm using biomarker guided therapy in Felker's paper and a 24 % reduction in the meta-analysis reported by Porapakkham [53]. Presumably the use of these markers emboldened the physician and/or the patient to increase the dose of ACE or ARB, aldosterone antagonist and/or beta blocker therapy. The studies targeting biomarker guided therapy did not demonstrate an improvement in the outcomes for patients over the age of 75. Thus if one adopts this approach and follows these markers to guide therapy in the clinical arena, it should probably be limited to patients below the age of 75 [54].

Elevated troponin concentrations in acute heart failure in the absence of a myocardial infarction or ischemia have been observed even in patients without underlying CAD. The presence of troponin in the blood is consistent with myocyte injury and/or necrosis and may help explain the poor prognosis associated with recurrent heart failure decompensations. In the ADHERE registry patients with a positive troponin had an 8.0 % mortality versus those without detectable troponin whose mortality was 2.7 % (P < 0.001) [55]. In addition, an elevated troponin in the outpatient setting is a marker of a worse prognosis [56] with higher mortality and morbidity for both the patient with acute as well as chronic HF.

Uric acid is an inexpensive, readily available and easily measured blood test that can serve as a biomarker of impaired oxidative metabolism and cytokine activation. These factors adversely impact the course of CHF. A metabolic, functional and hemodynamic (MFH) score has been proposed and subsequently validated [57, 58]. Uric acid is a powerful, independent predictor of prognosis in patients with HF. A serum level of ≥9.5 mg/dl correlates with 1 and 2 year mortality rates of 48 and 64 % versus 8 and 14 % for patients with uric acid levels below this value (P < 0.001). Uric acid alone was found to be as predictive as the HFSS in the group of patients studied.

Uric acid level ≥9.5 mg/dl, left ventricular ejection fraction ≤25 % and maximal oxygen consumption on stress testing of ≤14 cc O2/kg/min are each given 1 point. These values are summed to calculate the MFH score which ranges from 0 to 3. A score of 0 defines a low risk group with predicted 1 and 3 year mortality rates of 2 % and 9 % respectively. The 1 year mortality rates for scores of 1 and 2 are 23 % and 36 % respectively. A score of 3 identifies a very high risk group with a mortality rate of 69 % at 1 year and 88 % at 1.5 years.

How to Determine Who to Send for Advanced Options During the Transition of Care Phase

In hospitalized or ambulatory patients suffering with HF there are several factors useful in identifying those patients in need of advanced therapies. Patients with persistent NYHA Class

III-IV symptoms should be referred electively and this referral becomes urgent in cases where there is a concern for low output heart failure, the presence of refractory congestion or dysfunction of the kidneys or liver. Patients requiring a reduction in the dose of beta-blockers, ACE or ARB therapy due to symptoms or those with persistently low systolic blood pressure below 90–100 mmHg represent another high risk group. Any patient intolerant of beta-blockers or those exhibiting persistent tachycardia should be referred since the presence of an elevated heart rate is associated with a worse prognosis even in patients treated with beta-blockers [59–61]. Though not yet in the national guidelines for the management of congestive heart failure one should consider adding ivabradine in these cases. In the SHIFT trial ivabradine when added to GDMT resulted in a 26 % reduction in deaths from heart failure and a 26 % reduction in heart failure admissions.

Echocardiography helps the physician define the high risk patient who should be referred for advanced options. Findings of a markedly dilated left ventricle on ECHO (LVEDD >7.5 cm), increased left ventricular volume index (>120 cc/m^2), restrictive physiology, deceleration time ≤150 ms and mitral regurgitation vena contract width >0.4 cm have all been associate with a higher mortality rate [62]. Advanced right ventricular dysfunction defined as RVEF <20 % measured by nuclear ventriculography [63], ECHO features of right ventricular dysfunction including fractional shortening <32 %, right ventricular shortening <1.2 cm, tricuspid annular plane systolic excursion <1.4 cm and right ventricular annular tissue doppler index <10.8 cm/s have all been associated with an increase in mortality as well [64].

Persistent hyponatremia reflects excessive stimulation of the RAAS and is recognized as a major risk factor for adverse cardiovascular events as is any level of renal dysfunction [65]. One should also send any patient failing to respond to cardiac resynchronization therapy or experiencing ICD discharges, appropriate or inappropriate for referral as these all are associated with a poor prognosis. Additional high risk patients are those with a 6 min walk test distance of <300 m [66] or cardiopulmonary stress test demonstrating a VE/VCO2 slope >34 or a significant reduction in the peak oxygen consumption (provided anaerobic threshold obtained) defined as <12–14 cc O2/kg/min or <50–55 % predicted for age [67–69].

Patients who remain hemodynamically unstable during a hospitalization should be immediately transferred to a center capable of performing advanced heart failure therapies such as left ventricular assist device implantation and cardiac transplantation. Some of these patients may require support systems beyond intravenous inotropes and intra-aortic balloon counter pulsation (IABP) not routinely available in community hospitals. These devices include external corporal membrane oxygenation (ECMO), Tandem Heart and Impella 2.5, CP and 5.0 support systems. At our institution [INSERT REFERENCE] [70] we have enjoyed success using an Impella 5.0 device inserted surgically via the right axillary artery to reverse cardiogenic shock. This device is used as a bridge to the implantation of a durable left ventricular assist device or cardiac transplantation. We have found that using this method of support allows for recovery and/or improvement in the nutritional and functional status of the patient as well as hepatic and renal function. An axillary access allows the patient to remain mobile and capable of participating in a physical rehabilitation program.

Initiating a Palliative Care Discussion: An Important Step in the Transition to Outpatient Care

Once a patient has developed symptoms of stage D heart failure their mortality rate exceeds 50 % at 1 year. These patients have marked symptoms at rest and typically exhibit evidence of end organ hypoperfusion. In an effort to keep them comfortable or out of the hospital they require advanced options such as intravenous inotropes, circulatory support systems and/or cardiac transplantation. All stage D patients should undergo a palliative care discussion.

Planning for death is part of life and having a discussion with one's physicians and loved ones is as important as enacting a financial plan, a will or purchasing life insurance. Unfortunately, many people do not think of this and do not have these discussions with those closest to them before they become seriously ill. It is incumbent in such cases for the physician and the health care team to remind the patient of the importance of having these discussions and to assist the patient and those of their choosing with the information required to facilitate this effort. Due to the variable nature of CHF many physicians find a palliative care discussion daunting or fear that it may be emotionally taxing for the patient and family. The author has found that presenting this discussion as a "what if" scenario should the patient fail to respond to therapy is an effective way to introduce this topic. It is also important to assure the patient and the family that having this discussion is not an indication that there is no hope or that one is surrendering to the disease process. Instead it is simply an opportunity for the patient to reflect on their wishes in the event that their functional status declines to the point that they become incapacitated by their illness.

The opportunity to articulate their goals of care at that point to their loved ones is instrumental in the long-term care of these patients. As circumstances evolve the patient's desires will likely change over time and thus the palliative care plan should be updated. In so doing the patient's care choices are known to both his physicians and loved ones. This not only assures that the patients' wishes are honored but shields the loved ones from having to make emotionally difficult, trying and sometimes contentious decisions in an attempt to guess what the patient would want.

If a patient has NYHA Class IV symptoms despite GDMT and is not a candidate for advanced heart failure options then palliative care options should be discussed. Palliative care with continuous infusion of an inotrope may improve symptoms at the expense of shortening survival. This should be discussed with the patient as many are willing to accept this outcome. Since there is no data to support the contention that an ICD improves survival in these patients, one should not feel that the ICD must remain active or that one has to be placed in such patients if not already present or replaced if the generator reaches end of life. In fact, whether or not an inotrope is added at this time, the physician must discuss deactivation of the ICD and do not resuscitate orders for the hospital and ambulance/emergency transport vehicles in all of these cases.

Palliation means to ease symptoms without curing the underlying disease process. While code status certainly is addressed in a palliative care encounter, the topics discussed are much broader and extremely important in the care of a patient with congestive heart failure. The author believes that a discussion of the patient's wishes should occur early in the course of this disease, i.e., stage C due to the variable course many of these patients demonstrate and the high morbidity and mortality associated with CHF. When having this discussion with the patient they should be encouraged to include any loved ones, friends, religious associates or advisors that they would like to participate. It is important to realize that the patient is likely to consult with or lean on these sources for emotional and physical support as well as counsel over the coming days, weeks, months or even years.

It is appropriate to remind the patient to identify someone to make decisions on their behalf if they become incapacitated by enacting a medical power of attorney. Ideally, this person should be present for most if not all of the palliative care discussions. In cases where this is not possible a telephone conference call with all parties is encouraged. One should remind the patient that a medical and financial power of attorney is not the same legal document so that execution of the appropriate legal documents can be accomplished. Simple forms or a note signed by the patient and witnessed by an independent party is sufficient to declare this designation in most instances. If in doubt, one should always consult with an attorney to assure that the appropriate format is utilized. Many hospitals have legal staff available to assist the patient and physician in these matters.

Hospice Care for CHF Patients

Hospice should be discussed for patients with an estimated survival of <50 % at 6 months. Hospice agencies and the payors of these services must recognize the variability in the course of patients with CHF. As a result, our ability to distinguish between 50 % survival at 6 months versus 12 months is not always reliable. It is important to explain to the patient and family that the role of hospice is to keep one comfortable at home and to forego life sustaining care in the hospital setting. Instead, this care is replaced with compassionate comfort care in the home.

It is critical that one not forget to discuss the deactivation of an ICD in patients with end-stage heart disease as well as those patients suffering with terminal non-cardiac diseases such as cancer [71–75]. This should definitely be done by the time a patient reaches Stage D CHF if advanced options are not pursued.

It has been reported that only 50 % of patients entering hospice care with an ICD have the device deactivated. This omission can be particularly disturbing to both the patient and the family when the device fires postponing the death and prolonging the misery of the patient. Deactivation simply means discontinuing anti-tachycardia pacing and defibrillation. It does not require inactivation of either bi-ventriuclar pacing or bradycardia pacing modalities. This author routinely informs patients when discussing the implantation of an ICD that they can elect to inactivate the device at any time should their cardiac or general health condition change such that they would no longer want this resuscitative capability. This preparation makes any subsequent discussion of deactivating the device less traumatic for everyone.

Heart Failure Management Programs and the Transition of Care

Transitioning care from the in-patient to the outpatient environment is one of the most critical tasks facing physicians and hospitals caring for patients diagnosed with CHF. The 2013 Guideline for the Management of Heart Failure: A report of the American College of Cardiology Foundation/American Heart Association Task Force on Practice Guidelines, list the following recommendations for coordinating care for patients with chronic heart failure. Class I recommendations are:

1. Effective systems of care coordination with special attention to care transitions should be deployed for every patient with chronic heart failure that facilitate and ensure effective care that is designed to achieve GDMT and prevent hospitalization [76–93]. (Level of Evidence: B)
2. Every patient with HF should have a clear, detailed, and evidence based plan of care that ensures the achievement of GDMT goals, effective management of co-morbid conditions, timely follow-up with the healthcare team, appropriate dietary and physical activities, and compliance with Secondary Prevention Guidelines for cardiovascular disease. This plan of care should be updated regularly and made readily available to all members of each patient's healthcare team [94]. (Level of Evidence: C)
3. Palliative and supportive care is effective for patients with symptomatic advanced HF to improve quality of life [72, 95–98]. (Level of Evidence: B)

An institutional program for the management of heart failure is important to reduce readmissions and improve outcomes for CHF patients. The goals of such a program include implementing GDMT with the subsequent titration of these medications as an outpatient. In the hospital the patient and his caregivers should be educated on the disease as well as the myriad warning signs of incipient decompensated heart failure. It is critical that they understand these symptoms and report them to the care team. They should be instructed on the importance of weighing daily and recording the weights as opposed to trusting their memory. It is critical that along with the weights a journal recording any variations in diuretics necessitated by weight changes or symptoms be included. There should also be a record of all non-prescription and prescription medications on their person at all times and this should include documentation of when and why any medication was altered by themselves or anyone else. This log should be brought to each clinic visit along with the list of medications, all prescription bottles and any pill dispensers used by the patient for ready access and review by the healthcare team. This avoids conversations in the clinic regarding, "the small, round white pill or was it the yellow square one?," that invariably occur and is a source of frustration to the health care team as well as the patient. All instructions should be given verbally and reinforced in writing to assure the patient's comprehension as well as that of the caregiver.

In the hospital or clinic a program of "teach back" is helpful in those patients whose cognitive and physical condition allow. In this case the patient tells the nurse the name, dose, frequency and purpose of the medication. Allowing the patient to self administer medications in the hospital may also benefit future compliance. The hospital setting is the perfect place to stress the importance of daily weights, diet and if appropriate fluid restriction.

Ideally the patient should perform and record the daily weight with the supervision of the nursing staff. The author recommends that the patient bring their personal scale to the hospital. This allows one to confirm not only that they indeed have access to a reliable scale but also know how to zero and safely use this important tool in their home care. The patient is allowed to practice recording the weights and observe how the physician uses this information in their care, including the adjustments of diuretics. The patient and his caregiver should learn the orthodema scale discussed earlier and report worsening of this score even in the absence of a demonstrable weight gain.

One of the goals of treating heart failure is to maintain euvolemia using diuretics and dietary intervention to control symptoms and lessen hospitalization. Overly aggressive diuretic regimens can result in dizziness, dehydration, impairment of renal function, electrolyte disturbances, fatigue and lethargy. In some cases of severe HF, a fluid restriction must be implemented though it should not be recommended as part of the routine care of heart failure patients. When required, a reasonable oral fluid restriction should be prescribed. An oral allowance of 30 cc/kg for those weighing less than 85 kg and 35 cc/kg for those over 85 kg is reasonable [99, 100].

Sodium restriction is routinely advised though the data supporting this is generally poor. A sodium restriction of 5–8 g of table salt per day is a reasonable target. Tighter salt restrictions in conjunction with higher diuretic doses have been associated with higher rates of re-admission. Perhaps this is due to the development of diuretic resistance or stimulation of the RAAS and SNS. Research to guide physicians in this area is lacking and patient compliance with these efforts is generally poor [101].

A successful transition should also assure that co-existent medical conditions are optimally addressed and that the necessary arrangements are made for ongoing outpatient care. This includes evaluating and treating chronic kidney disease, anemia, thyroid disorders, diabetes mellitus, obesity, orthopedic and ambulatory issues, sleep apnea, depression as well as control of arrhythmias, ischemia, and hypertension.

The patient and caregiver should be questioned to assure that adequate resources are available to purchase medications and for follow-up physician care. If the patient does not possess these resources then consultation with a social worker is indicated to determine eligibility for national, state or local programs. At the time of discharge the patient and the caregiver should be given contact numbers to access providers and the support team via telephone 24 h a day, 7 days a week. An appointment within 3–7 days should be provided at the time of discharge to assure compliance and adjust therapies. Home health services may be of value in appropriate patients but are not an adequate replacement for physician care and clinic visits.

Monitoring Options to Consider as Part of a Heart Failure Disease Management Plan

Each institution and physician group will have to identify the most cost effective post discharge support that they can offer their patients. This could be something as simple as frequent clinic visits with self-reported weights. It is important to note that while the presence of weight gain over a couple of days is predictive of hospitalization for ADHF most patients hospitalized with ADHF do not experience a significant weight gain [102]. If these steps are not practical and/or additional resources are available one might consider adding telephone management by an office medical assistant, nursing staff, advanced practitioner or a clinical pharmacist.

A multi-disciplinary program targeting elderly patients with CHF achieved a 56 % reduction in heart failure admissions. However, this result is not proof of effectiveness since the primary endpoint of the trial, survival at 90 days without hospital readmission was negative [90]. The Specialized Primary and Networked Care in Heart Failure (SPAN-CHF) trial found a positive impact on 90 day readmissions by using nurses to visit and educate the patient at home followed by telephone contact once or twice a week to check on the patient, answer any questions and reinforce the education provided. Unfortunately this readmission benefit disappeared after the intervention ceased [103].

The DIAL (Randomized Trial of Phone Intervention in Chronic Heart Failure) study achieved a 20 % reduction in the combined endpoint of death or hospitalization 26.3 % versus 31.0 %, $P = 0.026$. The effect of the intervention was driven by a reduction in hospitalizations for HF, 16.8 % versus 22.3 % with no significant change in mortality. This improvement was likely due to the observation that at the end of the trial more patients in the intervention group were taking ACE, beta-blockers and aldosterone antagonists as well as diuretics and digoxin. In this trial nurses provided the intervention group with an educational booklet and performed phone calls every 2 weeks for 8 weeks though the frequency of the phone calls were adjusted based upon the nurses' assessment of the patients' needs. The improvement persisted for 3 years after the intervention was completed.

The results of the Telemonitoring to Improve Heart Failure Outcomes (Tele-HF) trial [104] utilizing telemonitoring failed to demonstrate a benefit from the intervention. In this study no improvement was observed in the combined end point of all cause hospital readmissions and all cause death rate nor was there any difference between the individual components of the primary end point. All of the secondary end points, hospitalizations for heart failure, number of hospitalizations or number of days in the hospital also failed to demonstrate a benefit of telemonitoring.

The Telemedical Interventional Monitoring in Heart Failure Study [105] enrolled ambulatory patients with NYHA Class II–III symptoms and a severely reduced LVEF ≤25 % or a LVEF ≤35 % in addition to a history of HF decompensation within 2 years. They were randomized to usual care versus telemedicine monitoring of weights, BP and ECG. The information was connected to a personal digital assistant and sent to the telemedicine system via an encrypted cell phone. This trial failed to demonstrate a difference in all cause mortality, cardiovascular death or HF hospitalizations at a median follow-up of 26 months.

The results of these telemonitoring trials support a cautious approach before one applies this strategy to all patients with CHF. Instead, one might wish to tailor an approach for the individual patient using these techniques in those whom the clinician feels might achieve the greatest benefit from such an intervention. This is especially prudent considering the mixed results demonstrating a lack of efficacy as it is unlikely that payors will reimburse physicians and hospitals for these services.

With the widespread use of ICDs in patients with CHF, companies have implemented various technologies to assist the clinician in an effort to detect clinically meaningful changes that may reliably detect the onset of ADHF. The goal was that early detection of adverse clinically silent events that predate the onset of ADHF would give the clinician time to implement an intervention thereby preventing an episode of ADHF resulting in hospitalization. Heart rate variability (HRV) is one such measure. It is derived from the pacemaker's ability to measure the intervals between successive atrial beats. HRV reflects the parasympathetic drive of the heart with higher degrees of HRV representing a greater influence of the parasympathetic system while loss of HRV reflects an increase in sympathetic drive which is seen in ADHF. Using a device based calculation known as the standard deviation of the atrial-to-atrial median (SDAAM) intervals one can predict the risk of hospitalization for ADHF as well as mortality [106]. An SDAAM of <60 ms compared to >100 ms was associated with a 3.2 fold increased 1 year mortality as well as higher risk of hospitalization. This parameter is useful in predicting long term events at 1 year as opposed short term events. There were changes in the SDAAM present within 3 weeks of a hospitalization for ADHF but the differentiation is too narrow to be of clinical use with current technology but if one observes a loss of SDAAM from baseline then it is reasonable to have the patient come to clinic for an assessment.

Intrathoracic impedance is reduced in the presence of fluid within the lung or pleural spaces. Using an ICD or pacing system allows measurement of the impedance between the lead tip and the pulse generator which should be superior to transthoracic measurements. Changes in impedance precede the onset of symptoms requiring hospitalization by an average of 18 days [107]. Clinical trials using this technology have been disappointing to date [108, 109]. There was one small study of 27 patients [110] that gives proponents of this technology hope for the future. However, at this time I would not recommend using these monitoring systems for the routine management of HF patients.

In the United States in 2015 the FDA approved the use of the CardioMEMMS device for reducing heart failure admissions in patients with both HFrEF and HFpEF. This is a wireless system implanted via the femoral vein into a branch of the left lower pulmonary artery. Data relaying the patient's pulmonary artery pressure is sent wirelessly to the monitoring center. The CardioMEMS Heart Sensor Allows Monitoring of Pressure to Improve Outcomes in NYHA Class III Heart Failure Patients, (CHAMPION) trial [111] was a single blinded study (patients blinded but not the physician) that evaluated this technology and noted a 30 % reduction in hospitalizations at 6 months associated with lower PA pressure measurements in the group receiving the implant. The group with the implant had observed changes in PA pressure addressed at the discretion of the treating physician independent of symptoms. This generally involved alterations in the doses of diuretic, ACE, ARB and/or hydralazine and nitrate medications. Outcomes were compared to the control group that was treated only on the basis of symptoms or clinical findings. A 28 % reduction in heart failure hospitalizations was observed over 6 months. This device was equally effective in reducing hospitalizations due to HFrEF as well as HFpEF.

Conclusion

The transition to outpatient care is critically important in the successful management of patients with CHF. The hospital physician must complete a detailed accounting of the hospital stay including the results of pertinent details of the history and physical exam and diagnostic tests. It is critical that the responsible physician assure that any diagnostic testing not performed in the hospital is performed expeditiously in the outpatient setting. GDMT must be adjusted and laboratory data collected as dictated by the circumstances of care.

A long-term management plan must be initiated during the hospitalization for ADHF. Using as the foundation the prognostic information obtained in the hospital the plan should be continually refreshed as additional information is acquired in the outpatient setting. Patients should be referred for device therapies and advanced therapeutic options as their condition and candidacy allows. Patient education of the disease process, medications, dietary restrictions and activity are critical. A palliative care discussion should be performed and a plan reflecting the personal wishes of the patient regarding the care of his disease documented with appropriate advanced directives.

A method to follow these patients with easy access to care must be assured. Ultimately the program chosen should assure the implementation of GDMT and a system to monitor the clinical status and function of the patient. The precise model one chooses is less important than adopting the aforementioned concepts to achieve cost-effective, high quality care. In so doing these patients will attain the best functional outcome and be afforded the best opportunity to improve their prognosis for one of the most deadly medical conditions in the world today.

References

1. Kociol RD, Hammill BG, Fonarow GC, et al. Generalizability and longitudinal outcomes of a national heart failure clinical registry (ADHERE) and non-ADHERE medicare beneficiaries. Am Heart J. 2010;160(5):885–92.
2. Jong P, Vowinckel E, Liu P, et al. Prognosis and determinants of survival in patients newly hospitalized for heart failure a population-based study. Arch Intern Med. 2002;162:1689–894.
3. Rosamond W, Flegal K, Fiday G, et al. Heart disease and stroke statistics-2007 update: a report from the American Heart Association Statistics Committee and Stroke Statistics Subcommittee. Circulation. 2007;115:e69–171.
4. Hunt SA, Abraham WT, Chin MH, et al. 2009 focused update incorporated into the ACC/AHA 2005 guidelines for the diagnosis and management of heart failure in adults: a report of the American College of Cardiology Foundation/American Heart Association Task Force on Practice Guidelines: developed in collaboration wit the International Society for Heart and Lung Transplantation. J Am Coll Cardiol. 2009;53:e1–90.
5. Owan TE, Hodge DO, Herges RM, et al. Trends in prevalence and outcome of heart failure with preserved ejection fraction. N Engl J Med. 2006;355:251–9.

6. Ceia F, Fonseca C, Mota T, et al. Prevalence of chronic heart failure in southwestern Europe: the EPICA study. Eur J Heart Fail. 2002;4:531–9.
7. Stewart S. Prognosis of patients with heart failure compared with common types of cancer. Heart Fail Monit. 2003;3:87–94.
8. Roger VL, Go AS, Lloyd-Jones DM, et al. Heart disease and stroke statistics-2012 update: a report from the American Heart Association. Circulation. 2012;125:e2–220.
9. Fang J, Mensah GA, Croft JB, et al. Heart failure related hospitalization in the U.S., 1979 to 2004. J Am Coll Cardiol. 2008;52: 428–34.
10. Braunstein JB, Anderson GF, Gerstenblith G, et al. Noncardiac co-morbidity increases preventable hospitalizations and mortality among medicare beneficiaries with chronic heart failure. J Am Coll Cardiol. 2003;42:1226–33.
11. Fonarow GC, Abraham WT, Albert NM, et al. Factors identified as precipitating hospital admissions for heart failure and clinical outcomes: findings from OPTIMIZE-HF. Arch Intern Med. 2008;168:847–54.
12. Bueno H, Ross JS, Wang Y, et al. Trends in length of stay and short term outcomes among medicare patients hospitalized for heart failure, 1993–2006. JAMA. 2010;303:2141–7.
13. Heidenreich PA, Sahay A, Kapoor JR, et al. Divergent trends in survival and readmission following a hospitalization for heart failure in the veterans affairs health care system 2002 to 2006. J Am Coll Cardiol. 2010;56:362–8.
14. Roccaforte R, Demers C, Baldassarre F, et al. Effectiveness of comprehensive disease management programmes in improving clinical outcomes in heart failure patients. A meta-analysis. Eur J Heart Fail. 2005;7:133–1144.
15. Phillips CO, Wright SM, Kern DE, et al. Comprehensive discharge planning with postdischarge support for older patients with congestive heart failure. A meta-analysis. JAMA. 2004;291:1356–67.
16. Heart Failure Society of America. The 2010 Heart Failure Society of America comprehensive heart failure practice guideline. Disease management, advance directives, and end of life care in heart failure: HFSA 2010 comprehensive heart failure practice guideline. J Card Fail. 2010;16:e98–114.
17. Gheorghiade M, Filippatos G, De Luca L, et al. Congestion in heart failure syndromes: an essential target of evaluation and treatment. Am J Med. 2006;19:s3–10.

18. Adams JF, Fonarow GC, Emerman CL, et al. Characteristics and outcomes of patients hospitalized for heart failure in the United States: rationale, design, and preliminary observations from the first 100,000 cases in the Acute Decompensated Heart Failure Registry (ADHERE). Am Heart J. 2005;149:209–16.

19. O'Connor CM, Stough WG, Gallup DS, et al. Demographics, clinical characteristics, and outcomes of patients hospitalized for decompensated hear failure: observations from the IMPACT-HF registry. J Card Fail. 2005;11:200–5.

20. Puligano G, DelSindaco D, Tavazzi L, et al. Clinical features and outcomes of elderly outpatients with heart failure followed up in hospital cardiology units: data from a large nationwide cardiology database (IN-CHF Registry). Am Heart J. 2002;143: 45–55.

21. Kao DP, Davis G, Aleong R, et al. Effect of bucindolol on heart failure outcomes and heart rate response in patients with reduced ejection fraction heart failure and atrial fibrillation. Eur J Heart Fail. 2013;15:324–33.

22. Lechat P, Julot JS, Escolano S, et al. Heart rate and cardiac rhythm relationships with bisoprolol benefit in chronic heart failure in CIBIS II trial. Circulation. 2011;103:1428–33.

23. van Veldhuisen DJ, Aass H, El Allaf D, et al. Presence and development of atrial fibrillation in chronic heart failure. Experiences from the MERIT-HF study. Eur J Heart Fail. 2006;8:539–46.

24. Joglar JA, Acusta AP, Shusterman NH, et al. Effect of carvedilol on survival and hemodynamics in patients with atrial fibrillation and left ventricular dysfunction: retrospective analysis of the US carvedilol heart failure trials program. Am Heart J. 2001;142:498–501.

25. Swedberg K, Komajda M, Bohm M, et al. Ivabradine and outcomes in chronic heart failure (SHIFT): a randomized placebo-controlled study. Lancet. 2010;376:875–85.

26. Levy D, Larson MG, Vasan RS, et al. The progression from hypertension to congestive heart failure. JAMA. 1996;275:1557–62.

27. Schocken DD, Benjamin EJ, Fonarow GC, et al. Prevention of heart failure: a scientific statement from the American Heart Association Councils on epidemiology and prevention, clinical cardiology. Cardiovascular nursing and high blood pressure research; quality of care and outcomes research interdisciplinary working group; and functional genomics and translational biology interdisciplinary working group. Circulation. 2008;117:2544–65.

28. Cooper LT, Baughman KL, Feldman AM, Frustaci A, Jessup M, Kuhl U, et al. The role of endomyocardial biopsy in the management of cardiovascular disease: a scientific statement from the American Heart Association, the American College of Cardiology, and the European Society of of Cardiology. Circulation. 2007;116:2216–23.
29. Fonarow GC, Adams KF, Abraham WT, et al. Risk stratification for in hospital mortality in acutely decompensated heart failure: classification and regression tree analysis. JAMA. 2005;293:572–80.
30. Hillege HL, Nitsch D, Pfeffer Ma, et al. Renal function as a predictor of outcome in a broad spectrum of patients with heart failure. Circulation. 2006;113:671–8.
31. Abraham WT, Fonarow GC, Albert NM, et al. Predictors of in hospital mortality in patients hospitalized with heart failure: insights from the Organized Program to Initiate Lifesaving Treatment in Hospitalized Patients with Heart Failure (OPTIMIZE-HF). J Am Coll Cardiol. 2008;52:347–56.
32. Gheorghiade M, Konstam MA, Burnett JC, et al. Short-term clinical effects of tolvaptan, an oral vasopressin antagonist, in patients hospitalized for heart failure: the EVEREST clinical status trials. JAMA. 2007;297:1332–43.
33. Konstam MA, Gheorghiade M, Burnett JC, et al. Effects of oral tolvaptan in patients hospitalized for worsening heart failure: the EVEREST outcome trial. JAMA. 2007;297:1319–31.
34. Ambrosy AP, Pang PS, Khan S, et al. Clinical course and predictive value of congestion during hospitalization in patients admitted for worsening signs and symptoms of heart failure with reduced ejection fraction: finding from the EVEREST trial. Eur Heart J. 2013;34:835–43.
35. Lala A, McNulty SE, Mentz RJ, et al. Relief and recurrence of congestion during and after hospitalization for acute heart failure. Circ Heart Fail. 2015;8:741–8.
36. Lucas C, Johnson W, Hamilton MA, et al. Freedom from congestion predicts good survival despite previous clas IV symptoms of heart failure. Am Heart J. 2000;140:840–7.
37. Rogers JG, Hellkamp AS, Young J, et al. Low congestin score 1 month after hospitalization predicts better function and survival. J Am Coll Cardiol. 2007;49:47A.
38. The ESCAPE Investigators and ESCAPE Study Coordinators. Evaluation study of congestive heart failure and pulmonary artery catheterization effectiveness. JAMA. 2005;294:1625–33.

39. Aronson D, Burger Aj, et al. Relation between pulse pressure and survival in patients with decompensated heart failure. Am J Cardiol. 2004;93:785–8.

40. Voors AA, Petrie Cj, Petrie Mc, et al. Low pulse pressure is independently related to elevated natriuretic peptides and increased mortality in advanced chronic heart failure. Eur Heart J. 2005;26:1759–64.

41. Stevenson LW, Perloff Jk, et al. The limited reliability of physical signs for estimating hemodynamics in chronic heart failure. JAMA. 1989;261:884–8.

42. Forrester JS, Diamond G, Chatterjee K, Swan HJ. Medical theapy of acute myocardial infarction by application of hemodynamic subsets (first of two parts). N Engl J Med. 1976;295: 1356–62.

43. Forrester JS, Diamond G, Chatterjee K, Swan HJ. Medical theapy of acute myocardial infarction by application of hemodynamic subsets (second of two parts). N Engl J Med. 1976;295: 1404–13.

44. Nohria A, Tsang B, Fang J, et al. Clinical assessment identifies hemodynamic profiles that predict outcomes in patients admitted with heart failure. J Am Coll Cardiol. 2003;41:1797–804.

45. Aaronson KD, Schwartz JS, Chen TM, et al. Development and prospective validation of a clinical index to predict survival in ambulatory patients referred for cardiac transplant evaluation. Circulation. 1997;95:2660–7.

46. Koelling TM, Joseph S, Aaronson KD. Heart failure survival score continues to predict clinical outcomes in patients with heart failure receiving beta-blockes. J Heart Lung Transplant. 2004;23:1414–22.

47. Levy WC, Mozaffarian D, Linker DT, et al. The seattle heart failure model: prediction of survival in heart failure. Circulation. 2006;113:1424–33.

48. Campana C, Gavazzi A, Beruni C, et al. Predictors of prognosis in patients awaiting heart transplantation. J Heart Lung Transplant. 1993;12:756–65.

49. Morrow D, de Lemos J. Benchmarks for the assessment of novel cardiovascular biomarkers. Circulation. 2007;115:949–52.

50. Braunwald E. Biomarkers in heart failure. N Engl J Med. 2008;358:2148–59.

51. Maisel AS, Krishnaswamy P, Nowak RM, et al. Rapid measurement of B-type natriuretic peptide in the emergency diagnosis of heart failure. N Engl J Med. 2002;347:161–7.

52. Januzzi JL, Camargo CA, Anwaruddin S, et al. The N-terminal pro-BNP investigation of dyspnea in the Emergency Department (PRIDE) study. Am J Cardiol. 2005;95:948–54.

53. Porapakkham P, Porapakkham P, Zimmet H, et al. B-type natriuretic peptide guided heart failure therapy a meta-analysis. Arch Intern Med. 2010;170:507–14.

54. Yancy Cw, Jessup M, Bozkurt B, et al. A report of the american college of cardiology foundation/american heart association task force on practice guidelines. J Am Coll Cardiol. 2013;62: e147–e239.

55. Peacock WF, De Marco T, Fonarow GC, et al. Cardiac troponin and outcome in acute heart failure. N Engl J Med. 2008;358:2117–26.

56. Hudson MP, O'Connor CM, Gattis WA, et al. Implications of elevated cardiac troponin T in ambulatory patients with heart failure: a prospective analysis. Am Heart J. 2004;147:546–52.

57. Anker SD, Coats AJS. Metabolic, functional, and haemodynamic staging for CHF? Lancet. 1996;348:1530–1.

58. Anker SD, Doehner W, Rauchlaus M, et al. Uric acid and survival in chronic heart failure; validation and application in metabolic, functional and hemodynamic staging. Circulation. 2003;107:1991–7.

59. Fox K, Ford I, Steg PG, et al. Heart rate as a prognostic risk factor in patients with coronary artery disease and left ventricular dysfunction (BEAUTIFUL): a subgroup analysis of a randomised controlled trial. Lancet. 2008;372:817–21.

60. Pocock SJ, Wang D, Pfeffer MA, et al. Predictors of mortality and morbidity in patients with chronic heart failure. Eur Heart J. 2006;27:65–75.

61. Flannery G, Gehrig-Mills R, Billah B, et al. Analysis of randomized controlled trials on the effect of magnitude of heart rate reduction on clinical outcomes in patients with systolic chronic heart failure receiving beta-blockers. Am J Cardiol. 2008;101:865–9.

62. Grayburn PA, Appleton CP, De Maria AN, et al. Echocardiographic predictors of morbidity and mortality in patients with advanced heart failure. J Am Coll Cardiol. 2005;45:1064–71.

63. Meyer P, Filippatos GS, Ahmed MI, et al. Effects of right ventricular ejection fraction on outcomes in chronic systolic heart failure. Circulation. 2010;121:252–8.

64. Grayburn PA, Appleton CP, Demaria AN, et al. Echocardiographic predictors of morbidity and mortality in patients with advanced heart failure the beta-blocker evaluation of survival (best). J Am Coll Cardiol. 2005;45:1064–71.
65. Smith GL, Lichtman JH, Bracken MB, et al. Renal impairment and outcomes in heart failure: systematic review and meta-analysis. J Am Coll Cardiol. 2006;47:1987–96.
66. Cahalin LP, Mathier MA, Semigran MJ, et al. The six minute walk test predicts oxygen uptake and survival in patients with advanced heart failure. Chest. 1996;110:325–32.
67. Mancini DM, Eisen H, Kussmaul W, et al. Value of peak exercise oxygen consumption for optimal timing of cardiac transplantation in ambulatory patients with heart failure. Circulation. 1991;83:778–86.
68. Arena R, Myers J, Aslam SS, et al. Peak VO2 and VE/VCO2 slope in patients with heart failure: a prognostic comparison. Am Heart J. 2004;147:354–60.
69. Balady GJ, Arena R, Sietsema K, et al. AHA scientific statement Clinician's guide to cardiopulmonary exercise testing in adults. Circulation. 2010;122:191–225.
70. Bansal A, Bhama Jk, Patel H, et al. Bridge to decision lvad support using the impella 5.0 Via a right subclavian artery approach. JHLT. 2013;32:S281.
71. Hauptman PJ, Swindle J, Hussain Z, Burroughs TE. Physician attitudes toward end stage heart failure: a national survey. Am J Med. 2008;121:127–35.
72. Hauptman PJ, Havranek EP. Integrating palliative care into heart failure care. Arch Intern Med. 2005;165:374–8.
73. Hauptman PJ. Palliation in heart failure: when less and more are more. Am J Hosp Palliat Care. 2006;23:150–2.
74. Goldestein NE, Lampert R, Bradley E, et al. Management of implantable cardioverter defibrillators in end of life care. Ann Intern Med. 2004;141:835–8.
75. Goldstein NE, Carlson M, Livote E, Kutner JS. Brief communication: management of implantable cardioverter-defibrillators in hospice: a nationwide survey. Ann Intern Med. 2010;152:296–9.
76. Inglis SC, Clark RA, McAlister FA, et al. Structured telephone support or telemonitoring programmes for patients with chronic heart failure. Cochrane Database Syst Rev. 2010;(8):CD007228.

77. McAlister FA, Stewart S, Ferrua S, et al. Multidisciplinary strategies for the management of heat failure patients at high risk for admission: a systematic review of randomized trials. J Am Coll Cardiol. 2004;44:810–9.
78. Naylor MD, Brooten DA, Campbell RL, et al. Transitional care of older adults hospitalized with heart failure: a randomized, controlled trial. J Am Geriatr Soc. 2004;52:675–84.
79. Coleman EA, Boult C. Improving the quality of transitional care for persons with complex care needs. J Am Geriatr Soc. 2003;51:556–7.
80. Stewart S, Pearson S, Horowitz JD. Effects of a home-based intervention among patients with congestive heart failure discharged from acute hospital care. Arch Intern Med. 1998;158:1067–72.
81. Stewart S, Marley JE, Horowitz JD. Effects of a multidisciplinary, home-based intervention on unplanned readmissions and survival among patients with chronic congestive heart failure: a randomised control study. Lancet. 1999;354:1077–83.
82. Sochalski J, Jaarsma T, Krumholz HM, et al. What works in chronic care management: the case of heart failure. Health Aff (Millwood). 2009;28:179–89.
83. Laramee AS, Levinsky SK, Sargent J, et al. Case management in a heterogeneous congestive heart failure population: a randomized control trial. Arch Intern Med. 2003;163:809–97.
84. Clark RA, Inglis SC, McAlister FA, et al. Telemonitoring of structured telephone support programmes for patients with chronic heart failure: systematic review and meta-analysis. BMJ. 2007;334:942.
85. Chaudhry SI, Phillips CO, Stewart SS, et al. Telemonitoring for patients with chronic heart failure: a systematic review. J Card Fail. 2007;13:56–62.
86. Riegel B, Carlson B, Kopp Z, et al. Effect of a standardized nurse case-management telephone intervention on resource use in patients with chronic heart failure. Arch Intern Med. 2002;162:705–12.
87. Riegel B, Carlson B, Glaser D, et al. Randomized controlled trial of telephone case management in Hispanics of Mexican origin with heart failure. J Card Fail. 2006;12:211–9.
88. Krumholz HM, Currie PM, Riegel B, et al. A taxonomy for disease management: a scientific statement from the American Heart Association disease management taxonomy writing group. Circulation. 2006;114:1432–45.

89. Faxon DP, Schwamm LH, Pasternak RC, et al. Improving quality of care through disease management: principles and recommendations from the American Heart Association expert panel on disease management. Circulation. 2004;109:2651–4.
90. Rich MW, Beckham V, Wittenberg C, et al. A multidisciplinary intervention to prevent the readmission of elderly patients with congestive heart failure. N Engl J Med. 1995;333:1190–5.
91. McAlister FA, Lawson FM, Teo KK, et al. A systematic review of randomized trials of disease management programs in heart failure. Am J Med. 2001;110:378–84.
92. Riegel B, LePetri B. Heart failure disease management models. In: Moser D, Riegel B, editors. Improving outcomes in heart failure: an interdisciplinary approach. Gaithersburg: Aspen Publishers Inc; 2001. p. 267–81.
93. Coleman EA, Mahoney E, Parry C. Assessing the quality of preparation for posthospital care from the patient's perspective: The care transitions measure. Med Care. 2005;43:246–55.
94. Smith SC, Benjamin EJ, Bonow RO, et al. AHA/ACCF secondary prevention and risk reduction therapy for patients with coronary and other atherosclerotic vascular disease: 2011 update: a guideline from the American Heart Association and American College of Cardiology Foundation. Circulation. 2011;124:2458–73.
95. Allen LA, Stevenson LW, Grady KL, et al. Decision making in advanced heart failure: a scientific statement from the American Heart Association. Circulation. 2012;125:1928–52.
96. Lorenz KA, Lynn J, Dy SM, et al. Evidence for improving palliative care at the end of life: a systematic review. Ann Intern Med. 2008;148:147–59.
97. Adler ED, Goldfinger JZ, Kalman J, et al. Palliative care in the treatment of advanced heart failure. Circulation. 2009;120:2597–606.
98. Qaseem A, Snow V, Shekelle P, et al. Evidence-based interventions to improve the palliative care of pain, dyspnea, and depression at the end of life: a clinical practice guideline from the American College of Physicians. Ann Intern Med. 2008;148:141–6.
99. Holst M, Stromberg A, Lindholm M, et al. Liberal versus restrictive fluid prescription in stabilized patients with chronic heart failure: result of a randomized cross-over study of the effects on health related quality of life, physical capacity, thirst and morbidity. Scand Cardiovasc J. 2008;42:316–22.

124   C.C. Eiswirth

100. Holst M, Stromberg A, Liindholm M, et al. Description of self reported fluid intake and its effects on body weight, symptoms, quality of life and physical capacity in patients with stable chronic heart failure. J Clin Nurs. 2008;17:2318–26.
101. Lainscak M, Blue L, Clark AL, et al. Self-care management of heart failure: practical recommendations from the Patient Care Committee of the Heart Failure Association of the European Society of Cardiology. Eur J Heart Fail. 2011;13:115–26.
102. Chaudhry SI, Wang Y, Concato J, et al. Patterns of weight change preceding hospitalizations for heart failure. Circulation. 2007; 116:1549–54.
103. Kimmelstiel C, Levine D, Perry K, et al. Randomized, controlled evaluation of short and long-term benefits of heart failure disease management within a diverse provider network: the SPAN-CHF trial. Circulation. 2004;110:1450–5.
104. Chaudhry SI, Mattera JA, Curtis JP, et al. Telemonitoring in patients with heart failure. N Engl J Med. 2010;363:2301–9.
105. Koehler F, Winkler S, Schieber M, et al. Impact of remote telemedical management on mortality and hospitalizations in ambulatory patients with chronic heart failure. Circulation. 2011;123:1873–80.
106. Adamson PB, Smith AL, Abraham WT, et al. Continuous autonomic assessment in patients with symptomatic heart failure: prognostic value of heart rate variability measured by an implanted cardiac resynchronization device. Circulation. 2004;110:2389–94.
107. Yu CM, Wang L, Chau E, et al. Intrathoracic impedance monitoring in patients with heart failure: correlation with fluid status and feasibility of early warning preceding hospitalization. Circulation. 2005;112:841–8.
108. Vollman D, Nagele H, Scharerte P, et al. Clinical utility of intrathoracic impedance monitoring to alert patients with an implanted device of deteriorating chronic heart failure. Eur Heart J. 2007;28:1835–40.
109. Ypenburg C, Bax JJ, van der Wall EE, et al. Intrathoracic impedance monitoring to predict decompensated heart failure. Am J Cardiol. 2007;99:554–7.
110. Maines M, Catanzariti D, Cemin C, et al. Usefulness of intrathoracic fluid accumulation monitoring with an implantable biventricular defibrillator in reducing hospitalizations in patient with heart failure: a case–control study. J Interv Card Electrophysiol. 2007;19:201–7.
111. Abraham WT, Adamson PB, Bourge RC, et al. Wireless pulmonary artery hemodynamic monitoring in chronic heart failure: a randomized controlled trial. Lancet. 2011;377:658–66.

Chapter 4
Volume Assessment and Management: Medical and Device Therapies

Lauren B. Cooper and Robert J. Mentz

Introduction

The clinical syndrome of heart failure is a constellation of signs and symptoms resulting from a reduced ability of the heart to pump an adequate volume of blood, either due to impaired ventricular filling or impaired ventricular pumping [1]. Heart failure patients retain sodium and fluid and may develop congestive symptoms of dyspnea, fatigue, and peripheral edema. Congestion is associated with increased morbidity and mortality in heart failure patients. Thus, the clinician should routinely assess clinical congestion based on history and physical examination. In addition, laboratory and imaging modalities as well as more recently developed implantable device technologies may assist with the diagnostic evaluation of congestion. The management of congestion has historically been based on loop diuretics, however, additional pharmacologic therapies such as thiazide diuretics, vasodilators, vasopressin antagonists, and mineralocorticoid receptor antagonists may provide additional decongestion

L.B. Cooper, MD (✉) • R.J. Mentz, MD
Division of Cardiology, Department of Medicine,
Duke University Medical Center, Durham, NC, USA
e-mail: Lauren.B.Cooper@duke.edu

H.O. Ventura (ed.), *Pharmacologic Trends of Heart Failure*, 125
Current Cardiovascular Therapy,
DOI 10.1007/978-3-319-30593-6_4,

benefits. If diuretic-based therapies are unsuccessful, ultrafiltration may be considered. In this chapter, we review the assessment of clinical congestion and highlight recent device-based diagnostic technologies. The approach to volume management is outlined including both pharmacologic and mechanical fluid removal.

Epidemiology of Congestion

Heart failure is a considerable and costly public health problem in the United States and worldwide, affecting more the 5 million American adults, responsible for over 1 million hospitalizations and costing over $30 million in 2012 [2]. Most heart failure hospitalizations are due to volume overload, with adequate decongestion therefore a major goal during hospitalization [3]. Despite inpatient treatment, many patients are discharged with persistent congestion, and congestion at the time of discharge is associated with worse outcomes [3–5]. Therefore, adequate assessment and treatment of volume overload are important factors in the management of patients with heart failure.

Terminology and Pathophysiology of Congestion

First described by Starling in 1914, as the normal heart fills with blood during diastole, the filling pressure in the ventricle increases, and the resultant stroke volume increases proportionally [6]. In heart failure, the ventricle is unable to increase stroke volume, either due to impaired contraction, impaired relaxation, or both (Fig. 4.1). Typically, during diastole the ventricle can accommodate large increases in volume with small increases in pressure. However, as the ventricle fills to capacity and becomes less distensible, the result is a significant rise in end-diastolic pressure. Therefore, the ventricular end-diastolic pressure is a marker of volume status. Congestion, or volume overload, in the setting of left ventricular dysfunction

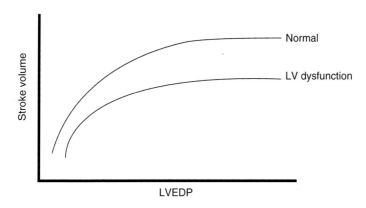

FIGURE 4.1 Starling curve. The relationship between stroke volume and left ventricular end-diastolic pressure in the setting of normal cardiac function and left ventricular dysfunction

is defined in part based on high left ventricular end diastolic pressure (LVEDp). LVEDp can be measured directly with a catheter passed retrograde through the aortic valve into the left ventricle or estimated via indirect measurements with a pulmonary artery catheter. In the absence of mitral valve disease, the left atrial pressure (LAp) is equal to the LVEDp, and the pulmonary capillary wedge pressure (PCWP) is a surrogate for the LAp and therefore for the LVEDp.

The mechanisms of congestion in heart failure are thought to be a result of neurohormonal activation of the renin-angiotensin-aldosterone system as well as increased circulating levels of vasopressin (Fig. 4.2). Volume overload may occur in isolation, or in conjunction with decreased cardiac output. Causes of congestion and worsening cardiac function can vary and may be multifactorial. Possible precipitating factors including ischemia, infection, hypertension, arrhythmia, and dietary or medication noncompliance [7]. Another proposed mechanism is that a reservoir of blood from the splanchnic circulation gets abnormally distributed to the effective circulating blood volume in the presence of an abnormal hormonal milleau, as occurs in heart failure [8]. Congestion leads to further neurohormonal activation, and

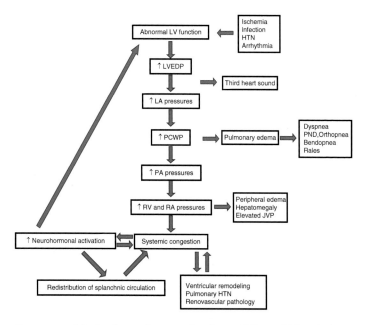

FIGURE 4.2 Mechanisms of congestive heart failure. Abbreviations: *HTN* hypertension, *JVD* jugular venous distension, *LA* left atrial, *LV* left ventricular, *LVEDP* left ventricular end diastolic pressure, *PA* pulmonary artery, *PCWP* pulmonary capillary wedge pressure, *PND* paroxysmal nocturnal dyspnea, *RA* right atrial, *RV* right ventricular

results in ventricular remodeling, pulmonary hypertension, and renovascular pathology, all of which contribute to worsening heart failure [9, 10].

Volume Assessment

History and Physical Examination

Symptoms

The clinical assessment can provide important information regarding volume status (Table 4.1). Patient reported

TABLE 4.1 Signs and symptoms of volume overload

Symptoms/signs	Etiology/hemodynamics
Left sided	
Dyspnea	Fluid accumulation in the lungs causing reduced lung compliance
Orthopnea (dyspnea when supine)	Increased ventricular preload: ≥2 pillows is consistent with a pulmonary capillary wedge pressure ≥28 mmHg
Paroxysmal nocturnal dyspnea	Fluid shifts from peripheral circulation
Bendopnea (dyspnea when bending)	Increasing right and left sided filling pressures
Rales	Pulmonary edema
3rd heart sound	Rapid ventricular filling during diastole
Right sided	
Edema	Increased venous pressures causing fluid to shift to interstitium
Hepatomegaly	Elevated right-sided filling pressures
Jugular venous distension	Elevated right atrial pressure
Bendopnea (dyspnea when bending)	Increasing right and left sided filling pressures

symptoms of congestion include dyspnea, dyspnea on exertion, orthopnea, paroxysmal nocturnal dyspnea, bendopnea, and edema [11].

The symptom of dyspnea is frequently reported by patients, and is one of the most common reasons they seek treatment for heart failure. Cardiogenic dyspnea is caused by fluid accumulation in the lungs that reduces lung compliance. Pulmonary edema is a result of high pressure in the pulmonary capillaries causing transudation of fluid into the alveolar walls and the alveolar spaces [12]. In the early stages of volume overload, dyspnea may only occur with exertion, but as congestion worsens, dyspnea can occur with progressively less exertion and even occur at rest. Shortness of breath may also present suddenly, as in "flash pulmonary edema," caused by acute increases in LVEDp caused by acute ischemia, acute aortic or mitral regurgitation, or severe hypertension. While the symptom of dyspnea is neither sensitive nor specific for volume overload, it can be used to subjectively assess response to therapy and characterize a patient's clinical course.

Orthopnea—dyspnea when supine—is due to the changes in blood distribution to the pulmonary circulation and increased ventricular pre-load when lying flat. Patients may describe this symptom in terms of the number of pillows required to sleep without experiencing shortness of breath. More severe orthopnea has been shown to correlate with higher pulmonary capillary wedge pressures [13]. A related symptom that occurs in the supine position is paroxysmal nocturnal dyspnea (PND). PND is acute shortness of breath that awakens a patient from sleep and results in an urge to sit upright and breathe cool air. PND is also thought to occur due to fluid shifting from the peripheral circulation.

Bendopnea—dyspnea when bending over—occurs when there are elevated right- and left-sided cardiac filling pressures. Compared to patients without bendopnea, patients with bendopnea have higher supine right atrial and pulmonary capillary wedge pressures, and both right and left sided filling pressures increase when bending over [14].

Physical Exam

Physical exam signs of congestion include peripheral edema, hepatomegaly, a third heart sound, rales, and jugular venous distention. Jugular venous distention and pulmonary rales are the most specific findings, and a third heart sound is the most sensitive finding [11].

Peripheral edema is the result of high right heart filling pressures which increases hydrostatic pressure in the venous circulation, causing fluid to shift into interstitial tissues. Like many signs and symptoms, the exam finding of dependent edema is not sensitive, but can be used to monitor response to treatment [11]. In addition to edema, marked elevation in right-sided filling pressures can also result in congestion of the liver, causing the liver to be enlarged and pulsatile. Prolonged congestive hepatopathy can result in irreversible liver damage, termed cardiac cirrhosis.

A third heart sound, termed an S3 gallop, is caused by rapid ventricular filling during the passive ventricular filling in diastole. The presence of an S3 is associated with elevated left atrial and left ventricular end diastolic pressures and is associated with a poor prognosis. As filling pressures decrease with diuresis, the S3 may diminish.

Pulmonary rales are due to fluid accumulation in the alveoli due to transudation of fluid due to increased pressures in the pulmonary veins. Volume overload causes elevated pressure in the left ventricle which leads to elevated pressures in the left atrium and pulmonary veins. While rales on the examination of the lungs may be heard, this finding can be found with other conditions. Additionally due to a compensatory increase in lymphatic drainage from the lungs in chronic heart failure, rales are often notably absent in many chronic heart failure patients despite significant patient-reported dyspnea [15].

Jugular venous pressure reflects right atrial pressure which typically correlates with pulmonary capillary wedge pressure. However, in approximately 20 % of patients, right atrial pressure and PCWP are discordant, with low RA pressure despite elevated PCWP, or, less commonly, high RA pressure despite low or normal PCWP [16, 17]. Therefore, JVP assessment is an important component of the evaluation of volume status in heart failure patients, but this should not be used in isolation.

Despite low sensitivity and specificity of individual patient-reported symptoms and physical exam findings, taken together, health care providers are commonly able to use these findings to diagnose decompensated heart failure, distinguish it from other disease processes and characterize the severity of congestion. Furthermore, changes in symptoms and exam findings can aid both patients and health care providers in monitoring volume status and response to therapy. Physician assessment of hemodynamics has been shown to correlate with invasive hemodynamic measurements, with clinical findings of congestion correlating with higher PCWP by invasive hemodynamic measurements [18].

Pulmonary Artery Catheters

In addition to noninvasive evaluations, pulmonary artery (PA) catheters can aid in the evaluation and monitoring of volume status. The Evaluation Study of Congestive Heart Failure and Pulmonary Artery Catheterization Effectiveness (ESCAPE) trial, studied heart failure patients hospitalized with congestion, and compared therapy tailored by clinical assessment versus invasive hemodynamic monitoring [13]. In this study, 433 patients were randomized to one of the two strategies with an endpoint of resolution of clinical congestion. While the trial did not show a difference in survival or hospitalization between patients who were treated with the aid of a PA catheter and those who were treated based on clinical assessment alone, the patients whose diuresis was adjusted based on the invasive hemodynamics had greater diuresis and less renal dysfunction with therapy [13, 19]. Furthermore, a review of patients excluded from the trial confirmed they were often more severely decompensated than those included in the trial [20]. Because physical exam findings can be confounded by factors such as discordant hemodynamics or valvular disease, PA catheters are recommended for patients with uncertain clinical pictures such as those with symptoms out of proportion to clinical exam findings and those not responding to therapy as expected based on clinical assessment alone [21].

Biomarkers: Natriuretic Peptides

Serum biomarkers, most notably the natriuretic peptides, can also be used to assess volume status and differentiate between signs and symptoms caused by heart failure versus other etiologies.

Brain Natriuretic Peptide (BNP)

Natriuretic peptides are neurohormones involved in natriuresis and diuresis. Brain natriuretic peptide (BNP) was originally identified in the brain, but is primarily released from the cardiac ventricles in response to volume overload and cardiac wall stress. Pre-proBNP is synthesized in the myocardium, cleaved first to pro-BNP, then cleaved to the biologically active BNP and the inactive NT-proBNP fragment. BNP causes myocardial relaxation and counteracts the effects of the renin-angiotensin-aldosterone system resulting in vasodilation, natriuresis, and diuresis [22].

In two prospective studies of patients presenting to the emergency department with complaints of dyspnea, the Breathing Not Properly (BNP) study and the N-terminal Pro-BNP investigation of dyspnea in the emergency department (PRIDE) study, natriuretic peptides were shown to accurately differentiate between dyspnea due to congestive heart failure versus dyspnea due to other causes [23, 24]. Elevated levels of BNP (>100 pg/mL) and NT-proBNP (>450 pg/mL for patients <50 years of age, >900 pg/mL for patients >50 years of age) were shown to have a high positive predictive value for shortness of breath due to congestive heart failure, while low levels of BNP (<50 pg/mL) and NT-proBNP (<300 pg/mL) had a high negative predictive value indicating dyspnea due to non-cardiac causes [23]. Furthermore, BNP and NT-proBNP levels were superior to other history, physical exam or laboratory findings for diagnosing acute heart failure [23–25].

BNP has been shown to correlate with high LVEDP, with decreases in BNP correlating with decreases in LVEDP [26, 27].

Furthermore, elevated BNP levels have been shown to correlate with heart failure severity and prognosis [24, 28, 29]. It is important to note, however, that BNP is influenced by a number of factors, with the elderly, females, and patients with renal dysfunction have been shown to have higher BNP levels, while obese patients typically have lower BNP levels [30–33]. It has been suggested that the change in BNP level for a particular patient compared to the baseline BNP or the admission BNP may be more accurate than the use of a fixed value for all patients [34]. Furthermore, BNP may not correlate with hemodynamics in patients with advanced heart failure [35], possibly due to changes in BNP clearance in patients with advanced disease [36]. Multiple studies with modest sample sizes have assessed the utility of using natriuretic peptides to guide therapeutic decisions in heart failure patients (Table 4.2). These studies have had variable results and a large-scale clinical trial, Guiding Evidence Based Therapy Using Biomarker Intensified Treatment (GUIDE-IT), is ongoing (clinicaltrials.gov, NCT01685840).

Atrial Natriuretic Peptide (ANP)

ANP is released from cardiomyocytes primarily in the atria. ANP has similar actions as BNP, acting as a vasodilator and increasing natriuresis and diuresis by reducing renal sodium reabsorption and decreasing the activity of the renin-angiotensin-aldosterone system [37, 38]. Despite the similarities, ANP has been shown to be inferior to BNP at predicting volume status and prognosis, and is therefore not used in the clinical setting [34].

Imaging

Chest Radiography

Chest radiographs can provide important clinical information and confirmation of physical exam findings for patients with heart failure and volume overload. The heart size can

TABLE 4.2 Summary of randomized controlled trials of biomarker guided therapy in heart failure

Trial name or first author	N	Marker	Target	Follow-up (months)	Primary endpoint	Results for primary endpoint
Troughton	69	NTproBNP	1692 pg/ml	9.6	CV death + CV hospitalization + worsening HF	+
STARS-BNP	220	BNP	100 pg/ml	15	HF death + HF hospitalization	+
TIME-CHF	499	NTproBNP	400 pg/ml (age <75) or 800 pg/ml (age ≥75)	18	All-cause death or hospitalization	Neutral
BATTLE SCARRED	364	NTproBNP	1270 pg/ml	12	All-cause death	Neutral
SIGNAL-HF	252	NTproBNP	50 % reduction	9	Days alive and out of hospital	Neutral
PRIMA	345	NTproBNP	D/C level	12	Days alive and out of hospital	Neutral

(continued)

TABLE 4.2 (continued)

Trial name or first author	N	Marker	Target	Follow-up (months)	Primary endpoint	Results for primary endpoint
Berger	278	NTproBNP	2200 pg/ml	15	Total days of HF hospitalization	+
STARBRITE	137	BNP	<2× D/C level	3	Days alive and out of hospital	Neutral
UPSTEP	279	BNP	150 ng/L (age <75) or 300 ng/L (age ≥75)	4	All-cause death + hospitalization + WHF	Neutral
PROTECT	151	NTproBNP	1000 pg/ml	10	Total CV events	+
GUIDE-IT	1100	NTproBNP		12	Time to CV death or first HF hospitalization	In progress

Abbreviations: *BNP* B-type natriuretic peptide, *CV* cardiovascular, *D/C* discharge, *HF* heart failure, *NTproBNP* N-terminal peptide fragment

be evaluated on chest imaging. Cardiomegaly, identified as the cardiac silhouette >50 % of the chest width, is an important clue in the diagnosis of new onset heart failure. Pulmonary findings including evidence of pulmonary hypertension, pulmonary edema, and pleural effusions can also aid in the assessment of patients with volume overload and are helpful in monitoring the efficacy of treatment for volume overload. Furthermore, chest radiographs can often identify other possible sources of the patient's symptoms.

Echocardiography

Echocardiography is considered the gold standard in identifying depressed ventricular function. Echocardiography is also a tool to assess volume status noninvasively. Size and respirophasic movements of the inferior vena cava (IVC) reflect right atrial pressure. Imaging of the inferior vena cava in the subcostal echocardiogram view can estimate right atrial pressure. A normal sized IVC of 1.5–2.5 cm diameter which collapses completely with inspiration corresponds to a right atrial pressure of 5–10 mmHg. Elevation of right atrial pressure leads to dilation of the vessel and loss of the normal inspiratory collapse. A nondilated IVC (1.5–2.5 cm) with <50 % collapse during inspiration corresponds to a right atrial pressure of 10–15 mmHg, and a dilated IVC (>2.5 cm) with <50 % collapse corresponds to a right atrial pressure of 15–20 mmHg. A dilated IVC of >2.5 cm with no respiratory collapse corresponds to a right atrial pressure of >20 mmHg [39]. As previously stated, right atrial pressure typically corresponds with pulmonary capillary wedge pressure, but can be discordant in some patients [16, 17].

Implantable Devices

Table 4.3 provides a summary of implantable fluid monitoring devices as well as several relevant clinical trials.

Table 4.3 Summary of trials of implantable fluid monitoring devices

Device name	Location/measurement	Study name	Trial design	Results
OptiVol (Medtronic)	Right ventricle/ Intrathoracic impedance	MID-HeFT	Prospective, observational, double-blinded N=33 NYHA Class III/IV	Correlation between impedance and PCWP: r = −0.61 (p<0.001) Correlation between impedance and fluid loss: r = −0.70 (p<0.001) Impedance decreases 15.3±10.6 days before symptom onset Detection of decreased impedance is 76.9% sensitive in detecting HFH with 1.5 false-positive detections per patient-year

FAST	Prospective, double-blind N = 156 NYHA Class I–IV	Comparison of changes in intrathoracic impedance (fluid index, FI) and changes in weight At 537 ± 312 days: Sensitivity for detection of HFE: FI 76.4 % vs Weight 22.5 %, (p < 0.001) Unexplained detection rate (changes in impedance NOT associated with an HFE) per patient-year: FI 1.9 vs Weight 4.3 (p < 0.001)

(continued)

TABLE 4.3 (continued)

Device name	Location/measurement	Study name	Trial design	Results
		DOT HF	Prospective, randomized, unblinded N = 335 (TG 168, CG 167) NYHA Class II-IV	Death or HFH at 14.9 ± 5.4 months: TG 29 % vs CG 20 % (p = 0.063)
Chronicle (MedTronic)	Right ventricle/RV pressure	COMPASS-HF	Prospective, randomized, single-blind N = 274 (TG 134, CG 140) NYHA Class III/IV	At 6 months: Freedom from DSC 92 % Freedom from DF 100 % HFE event rate: TG 0.67 vs CG 0.85 (p = 0.33)

HeartPOD (St. Jude)	Left atrium/LA pressure	HOMEOSTASIS	Prospective, observational, open label
			N = 40
			NYHA Class III/IV
				At 6 weeks:
				Freedom from MACE/MANE: 100 %
				Freedom from DF: 95 %
				Rate of HFE or death:
				  0.72 at 1 year
				  0.69 at 2 years
				  61 % at 3 years

CardioMEMS (CardioMEMS)	Pulmonary artery/PA pressure	CHAMPION	Prospective, randomized, single-blind n = 550 (TG 270, CG 280) NYHA Class III	At 6 months: Freedom from DSC: 98.6 % Freedom from DF: 100 % Rate of HFH:TG 0.32 vs CG 0.44 (p = 0.0002)

Abbreviations: HFH heart failure hospitalizations, *HFE* heart failure events (hospitalizations, ER visits, urgent clinic visits), *TG* treatment group, *CG* control group, *DSC* device or system complications, *DF* device failure, *MACE* major adverse cardiovascular events, *MANE* major adverse neurological events

Impedance Monitors

Another way to assess fluid status is through devices that measure intrathoracic impedance, which correlates with volume status. Electricity traveling between two points conducts better (i.e. decreased impedance) through water than through air (Fig. 4.3). As fluid accumulates in the lungs, the impedance across the lungs decreases [40, 41]. Devices that monitor impedance and record changes in impedance over time are included on some implantable cardioverter defibrillators.

OptiVol [42] (Medtronic, Inc., Minneapolis, MN) measures intrathoracic impedance between the tip of the right ventricular lead and the implanted device. The utility of the OptiVol device was studied in the Medtronic Impedance Diagnostics in Heart Failure Trial (MIDHeFT) [42], showing a decrease in intrathoracic impedance approximately 2 weeks prior to hospitalization for decompensated heart failure, and more than 1 week prior to the onset of symptoms. Furthermore,

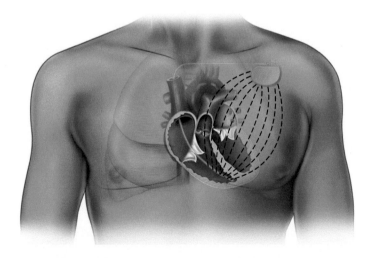

FIGURE 4.3 Measurement of intrathoracic impedance via an implantable device

with diuresis, there was a correlation with an increase in intrathoracic impedance. This concept was further tested in the Fluid Accumulation Status Trial (FAST) which showed that impedance monitoring was more sensitive than changes in weight for detecting fluid overload and worsening heart failure [43]. Additional studies have demonstrated that OptiVol monitoring can predict heart failure hospitalizations [44, 45], rehospitalizations [46, 47], and mortality [48]. However, when patients were given access to impedance information, via an automated alert for possible fluid accumulation, the result was more outpatient visits and hospitalizations, and no improvement in mortality compared with usual care [49]. OptiVol monitoring is currently available as a diagnostic feature on certain implantable defibrillators, and is being used as an additional diagnostic component in the overall volume assessment of patients.

While impedance monitors measure use algorithms to characterize volume status, there are also direct pressure sensors that can be implanted in the right ventricle, left atrium, or pulmonary artery.

Right Ventricular Pressure Monitor

Similar to an RV pacemaker lead, a right ventricular pressure monitor can be implanted in the right ventricle and continuously measure ventricular filling pressures [50]. The RV pressure monitor, Chronicle (Medtronic, Inc., Minneapolis, MN) was tested in the Chronicle Offers Management to Patients with Advanced Signs and Symptoms of Heart Failure (COMPASS-HF) study. While the hemodynamic data obtained from the device correlates with right heart catheterization data [51], compared to standard care, treatment with the Chronicle device did not reduce hospitalizations and it did not reduce emergency or urgent care visits requiring intravenous therapy [52]. In both the treatment group and the standard of care groups, there was a lower than expected event rate, which may have been due to regular and frequent contact with medical professionals which has previously been shown to improve heart failure outcomes [53, 54]. Thus, the role for RV pressure monitoring devices for the routine assessment of volume status in heart failure patients requires further study.

Left Atrial Pressure Monitor

A left atrial pressure monitor, the HeartPOD (St. Jude Medical Inc., Minneapolis, MN), measures left atrial pressure and is implanted surgically or transvenously via a transseptal puncture [55, 56]. In the Hemodynamically Guided Home Self-Therapy in Severe HF patients (HOMEOSTASIS) trial [57], the use of this device improved patient's functional status and ejection fraction, and allowed for up titration of heart failure medications and decreases in diuretic doses. The left atrial pressure monitor is currently being further studied in the Left Atrial Pressure Monitoring to Optimize Heart Failure Therapy (LAPTOP-HF) for safety and efficacy in reducing worsening heart failure and hospitalization (clinicaltrials.gov, NCT01121107). It will be necessary to demonstrate the efficacy of these devices to improve outcomes compared with current usual care prior to broad clinical application.

Pulmonary Artery Pressure Sensor

A pulmonary artery pressure monitor can be deployed in a pulmonary artery branch during right heart catheterization and provides accurate pulmonary pressure measurements [58]. A pulmonary artery pressure sensor, CardioMEMS (CardioMEMS, Atlanta, Georgia), was studied in the CardioMEMS Heart Sensor Allows Monitoring of Pressure to Improve Outcomes in NYHA Class III HF Patients (CHAMPION) trial [59, 60]. Use of this device resulted in a reduction in heart failure hospitalizations, pulmonary artery pressures, and an improvement in quality of life and medication utilization. The CardioMEMS device was approved by the FDA in October 2013.

The official practice guidelines for the management of heart failure recognize the advances in technology in the diagnostic evaluations of heart failure [21]. While initial studies suggest that implantable devices can provide accurate measurements that correlate with filling pressures, some of these devices are still being evaluated in larger clinical trials to determine the degree to which they impact outcomes. As these devices are adopted into routine clinical practice, they may be able to provide additional information in the evaluation of patients and the overall assessment of volume status.

Volume Management

Medical Therapy/Diuretics

Diuretics work by limiting sodium reabsorption in the kidney, resulting in increased urinary sodium and water excretion. The mechanism of action and the location of action in the kidney differ between classes of diuretics. Due to a positive charge, sodium can only cross the lipid luminal membrane into the cell by a transmembrane carrier or sodium channel. Sodium is transported out of the cell by Na-K-ATPase pumps in the basolateral cell membrane which return reabsorbed sodium to the systemic circulation. In the kidney, approximately 65–70 % of sodium is reabsorbed in the proximal tubule, 25 % is reabsorbed in the loop of Henle, and the remainder reabsorbed in the distal and collecting tubules [61]. Figure 4.4 presents the sites of diuretic action in the nephron.

Loop Diuretics

Loop diuretics include furosemide, torsemide, and bumetanide, and their mechanism of action is in the loop of Henle. The transmembrane carrier in the thick ascending limb of the loop of Henle is a Na+ K+ 2CL– cotransporter, which is dependent on chloride delivery. Loop diuretics compete for the chloride site on the transporter, thereby

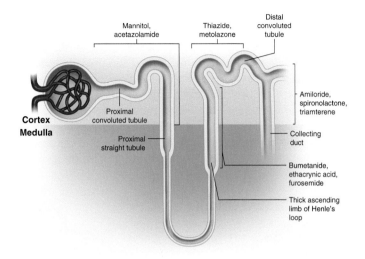

FIGURE 4.4 Sites of diuretic action in the nephron. Proximal tubular diuretics such as mannitol and acetazolamide, have a modest net negative effect on sodium balance because downstream nephron sites reabsorb much of the sodium that is not reabsorbed in the proximal tubule. Loop diuretics dose-dependently decrease sodium reabsorption in the thick ascending limb of the loop of Henle. Thiazides and metolazone inhibit sodium reabsorption in the early portion of the distal convoluted tubule. Triamterene, amiloride, and spironolactone are potassium-sparing diuretics that work at the late portion of the distal convoluted tubule and the cortical collecting duct. (Reproduced with permission)

limiting the transporter and blocking sodium reabsorption [62]. The pharmacology differs between the loop diuretics. Bumetanide and torsemide have a higher and more predictable bioavailability than furosemide. Torsemide has the longest half-life, but the half-lives of all of the loop diuretics increase with renal or hepatic dysfunction. The onset of action for loop diuretics is similar, 30–60 min if given orally and within minutes if given intravenously [63].

Loop diuretics are often the first line for treatment of volume overload in heart failure and are typically given intravenously in the setting of decompensation due to the need for a rapid onset of action. A pharmacologic review of loop diuretics highlights favorable outcomes in patients with heart failure treated with torsemide over furosemide, with respect to mortality, hospitalization, and functional class [63]. Additionally, in outpatients with heart failure, bumetanide has been shown to be more effective than furosemide at reducing dyspnea [64]. While continuous dosing of loop diuretics has theoretical advantages over intermittent bolus dosing, with a steady delivery of the drug to maintain a constant effect, the Diuretic Optimization Strategies Evaluation (DOSE) trial did not show a significant difference between the two approaches for the co-primary endpoints assessing patients' symptoms and creatinine change [65, 66]. The DOSE trial was a prospective, randomized trial to evaluate diuretic dosing strategies in patients hospitalized with decompensated heart failure. Three hundred eight patients were randomized in a 2×2 factorial design to IV furosemide given as twice daily boluses or continuous infusion, and to either low dose (equivalent dose to home dose) or high dose (2.5 times home dose). There was no significant difference between the bolus versus continuous infusion groups. However, compared to the low dose group, the high dose group had more favorable outcomes in terms of dyspnea relief, weight loss, and net fluid loss. The high dose group, however, had worsening renal function, though this was found to be transient and resolved by the 60-day follow up [65]. Thus, an evidence-based initial approach to congestion management involves high-dose intravenous diuretics, administered as bolus or continuous infusion dosing.

Thiazide Diuretics

Sequential nephron blockade with thiazide-type diuretics may be used in combination with loop diuretics to augment diuresis [67]. Thiazide diuretics including hydrochorothiazide, chlorothiazide, chlorthalidone, and metolazone, act in the distal tubule by inhibiting the Na+ Cl– cotransporter in this location. Because the distal tubule reabsorbs less sodium than the loop of Henle, thiazide diuretics are less potent than loop diuretics. However, if sodium is not absorbed proximally, as during administration of loop diuretics, there is a compensatory response for the excess sodium and water to be absorbed distally [62]. Under normal physiologic conditions, the distal tubule absorbs approximately 5 % of the filtered sodium; the capacity for reabsorption can more than double in response to increased flow to the distal tubule due to the effects of a loop diuretic [62]. Giving a thiazide diuretic in conjunction with a loop diuretic may increase effectiveness of the loop diuretic by preventing distal reabsorption of sodium [68]. Because thiazide diuretics have a longer half-life than loop diuretics, the effect on the distal tubule will continue even after the loop diuretic has worn off [67]. Thus, patients who take loop diuretics chronically may be instructed to take thiazide diuretics on an "as needed" basis for worsening volume overload, though this strategy has not been rigorously evaluated in a clinical trial. Furthermore, the use of thiazide diuretics has been associated with increased arrhythmia risk due to hypokalemia [69, 70].

Potassium Sparing Diuretics

Potassium sparing diuretics include sodium channel blockers and aldosterone antagonists. These groups of medications act at the collecting tubule via different mechanisms. In the collecting tubule, the luminal membrane contains sodium and potassium channels, not transporters. Sodium channel blockers, amiloride and triamterene, directly block the sodium channels in the luminal membrane.

Aldosterone acts as a diuretic by increasing the number of open sodium channels in the collecting tubule. In the setting of loop diuretic use, when sodium is not absorbed proximally in the loop of Henle, it can be absorbed distally via an upregulation of aldosterone-sensitive sodium channels in the collecting tubule. The aldosterone antagonists (also referred to as mineralocorticoid receptor antagonists [MRAs]), spironolactone and eplerenone, block the action of aldosterone resulting in decreased sodium reabsorption in the collecting tubule; therefore, the addition of an MRA to a loop diuretic may result in increased natriuresis and diuresis. Aldosterone antagonists are recommended for patients with heart failure and reduced left ventricular ejection fraction ≤35 % and New York Heart Association class II–IV symptoms, based on several studies which demonstrated a reduction in mortality in patients taking aldactone or eplerenone [71–73]. While the MRAs have both diuretic and potassium-sparing effects, they also offer additional cardiovascular benefits beyond these properties [74]. Heart failure patients taking only non-potassium sparing diuretics without concomitant use of a potassium-sparing diuretic have been shown to have an increased risk of progressive heart failure and death, likely due to deleterious effects of neurohormonal activation that occurs with diuretic use in heart failure [75, 76].

Diuretic Resistance and RAAS Activation

The efficacy of a diuretic depends on many factors: the dose of the drug, the rate of delivery of the drug to the renal tubule, and patient factors including sodium and fluid intake and co-morbidities including heart failure and renal dysfunction [62]. There is a dose response curve that differs between drugs and between oral and intravenous administration. A certain concentration of the drug is required before diuresis occurs. Once that threshold level is reached, the response increases with increasing dose of the drug. There is a ceiling on the dose responsiveness. Once the transporter or channel is saturated, the maximum rate of diuresis is reached, and further dose increases will not result in increased diuresis [62]. The goal with diuresis is to find an effective dose that results in an effect on the ascending portion of the dose-response curve (Fig. 4.5). In patients with heart failure, the dose response curve is shifted downward and to the right and patients become less responsive to diuretics, thus higher dose are often required to achieve effective diuresis [77]. While

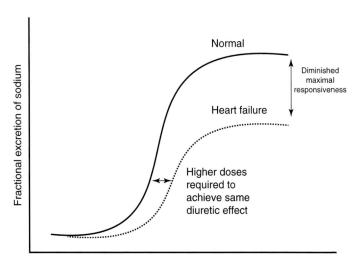

FIGURE 4.5 Dose response curve of loop diuretics. Schematic of dose-response curve of loop diuretics in heart failure patients compared with controls. In heart failure patients, higher doses are required to achieve a given diuretic effect and the maximal effect is blunted (Reproduced with permission from Felker [77])

some observational studies have shown an association between high dose loop diuretics and poor outcomes, these results are cofounded given that patients receiving higher doses of diuretics were likely more sick with more volume overload and possibly more diuretic resistance, requiring higher doses of diuretics to achieve a diuretic response [78].

Impaired renal function affects the bioavailability of diuretics. If the reduced glomerular filtration rate (GFR) is due to chronic kidney disease, there is impaired delivery of the drug to the kidney. A higher dose of the drug promotes an increased rate of delivery to the tubule and thus may be necessary in order to achieve efficacy in the setting of chronic kidney disease. If the reduced GFR is due to low cardiac output, improving hemodynamics can improve renal perfusion and diuretic efficacy [67]. Additionally, with volume overload resulting in intestinal edema, intestinal absorption of oral drugs may be impaired, therefore intravenous administration is preferred to overcome this issue [62].

In addition to adequately dosing and optimizing delivery of the drug, diuretic resistance may occur in patients being treated for volume overload. Several mechanisms contribute to diuretic resistance with loop diuretics: reduced diuretic efficacy with repeated dosing, rebound sodium retention due to increased sodium reabsorption in the distal nephron, and with chronic use, renal adaptation in the distal tubule resulting in hypertrophy and increased sodium reabsorption [66, 67]. One way to overcome diuretic resistance, in addition to increasing the dose of the drug, is to block sodium reabsorption in the distal tubule by giving a thiazide diuretic in conjunction with a loop diuretic (i.e., dual nephron blockade). However, treatment with combination diuretics can result in electrolyte disturbances, particularly hypokalemia, so electrolytes must be closely monitored and repleted during diuresis. Similarly, blocking downstream sodium reabsorption in the collecting tubule by administering an aldosterone antagonist can help overcome diuretic resistance. Reduced diuretic efficacy can be caused by neurohormonal activation, as diuretics may activate the renin-angiotensin-aldosterone system, which increases sodium reabsorption. This issue can be overcome with concomitant use of other medications that block the cascade, including ACE inhibitors, ARBs, and MRAs [67].

Vasopressin Receptor Antagonists

Vasopressin, or antidiuretic hormone, which is increased in the setting of heart failure has many systemic effects including vasoconstriction, cardiac hypertrophy, platelet aggregation, adrenocorticotropic hormone release, and uterine contraction [79]. Activation of the V2 receptor in the renal collecting tubule effects the aquaporin channels resulting in increased permeability to water which leads to water retention and hyponatremia [80]. Unlike diuretics that promote natriuresis and diuresis, vasopressin receptor antagonists, like tolvaptan, inhibit vasopressin, resulting in selective free water diuresis without natriuresis.

Treatment with tolvaptan has been shown to reduce weight, decrease dyspnea and edema, and normalize serum sodium levels in patients with hyponatremia [81–83]. Weight loss and symptom relief appears to be more significant in patients with hyponatremia. However, in heart failure patients, it has not yet been shown that treatment with tolvaptan improves long term mortality or cardiovascular morbidity [83]. Tolvaptan is approved for the treatment of severe or symptomatic hyponatremia in patients with heart failure.

Ultrafiltration

Ultrafiltration is an alternate strategy for volume removal. During the process of ultrafiltration, plasma water is removed from whole blood across a semipermeable membrane due to a pressure gradient across the membrane. Until recently, ultrafiltration has required central venous, but current devices allow for ultrafiltration through peripheral venous access [84]. In this technique, two peripheral intravenous catheters are placed, one for blood withdrawal and one for blood return, with ultrafiltration through a single-use extracorporeal blood circuit achieving fluid removal of up to 500 mL/h [66, 84]. Anticoagulation is typically required to prevent malfunction of the filter. Contraindications to ultrafiltration include hemodynamic instability, acute renal insufficiency, hypercoagulability, and poor venous access [66].

An advantage of ultrafiltration over diuretics is that ultrafiltrate is isotonic compared with urinary output with diuretics which is hypotonic. Thus, ultrafiltration removes more sodium and less potassium for the same volume compared with diuretics and may offer benefits related to maintain electrolyte balance [85]. Additionally, the rate of fluid removal can be titrated so that it does not does not exceed the interstitial fluid mobilization rate, preserving intravascular volume and avoiding the acute renal insufficiency the may occur with diuretic therapy [66, 86].

The first prospective, randomized, multicenter study comparing ultrafiltration with intravenous diuretic therapy in patients with heart failure and volume overload, the Ultrafiltration versus Intravenous Diuretics for Patients Hospitalized for Acute Decompensated Congestive Heart Failure (UNLOAD) trial, randomized 200 patients within 24 hours of hospital admission to either ultrafiltration or standard care with intravenous diuretics administered via continuous infusion or bolus injections [87]. At 48 hours, both groups had similar relief of dyspnea, but the ultrafiltration group had greater net fluid loss and greater weight loss. Both groups had similar length of hospital stay. At 90 days, the ultrafiltration group had fewer rehospitalizations and unscheduled clinic or emergency department visits. There were no differences in serum creatinine changes between the groups, and both groups had a similar number of deaths [87]. Further analysis comparing ultrafiltration to continuous intravenous diuretic therapy and to bolus intravenous diuretic therapy revealed similar degree of weight and fluid loss between the ultrafiltration and continuous infusion groups and between the continuous infusion and bolus dosing groups, but a greater degree of weight and fluid loss in the ultrafiltration group compared to the bolus dosing group [85]. However, despite similar weight and volume loss in the ultrafiltration and continuous infusion groups, there were fewer rehospitalizations and unscheduled visits to the clinic or emergency room in the ultrafiltration group [85]. Notably, the number of events was low and these findings warrant further validation in larger adequately powered studies.

Despite the favorable outcomes for ultrafiltration in patients with heart failure and volume overload, the outcomes may be different in patients with worsening renal function in the setting of decompensated heart failure and volume overload, as assessed in the Cardiorenal Rescue Study in Acute Decompensated Heart Failure (CARRESS-HF) study [88]. In this prospective randomized study, 188 patients with acute decompensated heart failure, worsening renal function with a rise in serum creatinine ≥0.3 mg/dL from baseline, and persistent congestion were randomized to ultrafiltration or a stepped pharmacologic therapy to maintain a urine output of 3–5 l/day. While the weight loss was similar between the groups at 96 h, the ultrafiltration group experienced a greater increase in serum creatinine. Furthermore, the ultrafiltration group had a higher rate of serious adverse events over the follow-up period of 60 days. At 60 days, there were no significant differences in weight loss, mortality, or rehospitalizations between the groups, and both groups had lower creatinine levels compared to baseline levels [88]. The difference in outcomes in these two trials highlights the complexity of implementing this novel technique to treat patients with volume overload. Current guidelines recommend consideration of ultrafiltration for relief of volume overload or for refractory congestion not responding to medical therapy [21].

Summary

Volume overload occurs in heart failure because of pathologic changes in hemodynamics and neurohormonal activation. Congestion is a major cause of morbidity and mortality in patients with heart failure, and thus it must be accurately recognized and adequately treated. The diagnosis of volume overload is often made based on patient and clinician assessments, though radiographic and echocardiographic findings and serum biomarker measurements can help confirm the diagnosis and monitor the effectiveness of treatment. Implantable devices to measure filling pressures are being developed and tested to provide additional information to incorporate into the overall clinical picture of congestion. Invasive hemodynamic monitoring can be pursued for cases in which noninvasive assessments are inadequate or confounded.

Treatment of volume overload consists of pharmacologic and mechanical strategies (Fig. 4.6) [89]. Diuretics increase urinary sodium and water excretion, with different classes of

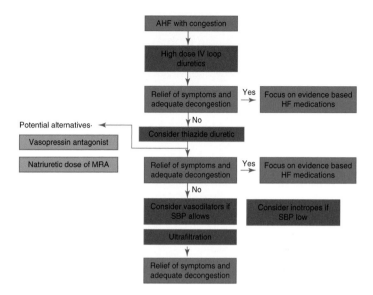

FIGURE 4.6 Management of volume overload in heart failure (Modified and reproduced with permission from Mentz et al. [89])

diuretics acting at different sites in the kidneys—loop diuretics at the loop of Henle, thiazide diuretics at the distal tubule, and potassium sparing diuretics and vasopressor receptor antagonists at the collecting tubule. When escalating doses of diuretics are ineffective, volume removal may be achieved with ultrafiltration, a process in which plasma water is removed from whole blood across a semipermeable membrane. Ultrafiltration, which once require central venous catheter placement, can now be performed through peripheral venous access.

Conclusions

Heart failure is a considerable public health problem worldwide. In this chapter, we reviewed the diagnosis and treatment of volume overload, one of the major sources of morbidity and mortality in heart failure. Despite the current assessment and management tools available to clinicians, the burden of heart failure remains high, highlighting the need for development of novel tools and strategies to improve outcomes in this patient population.

References

1. Braunwald E. Heart failure. JACC Heart Fail. 2013;1(1):1–20.
2. Mozaffarian D, Benjamin EJ, Go AS, et al. Executive summary: heart disease and stroke statistics-2016 update: a report from the American Heart Association. Circulation. 2016;133(4):447–54.
3. Gheorghiade M, Filippatos G, De Luca L, Burnett J. Congestion in acute heart failure syndromes: an essential target of evaluation and treatment. Am J Med. 2006;119(12 Suppl 1):S3–10.
4. Ambrosy AP, Pang PS, Khan S, et al. Clinical course and predictive value of congestion during hospitalization in patients admitted for worsening signs and symptoms of heart failure with reduced ejection fraction: findings from the EVEREST trial. Eur Heart J. 2013;34(11):835–43.
5. Lucas C, Johnson W, Hamilton MA, et al. Freedom from congestion predicts good survival despite previous class IV symptoms of heart failure. Am Heart J. 2000;140(6):840–7.
6. Patterson SW, Piper H, Starling EH. The regulation of the heart beat. J Physiol. 1914;48(6):465–513.
7. Schiff GD, Fung S, Speroff T, McNutt RA. Decompensated heart failure: symptoms, patterns of onset, and contributing factors. Am J Med. 2003;114(8):625–30.
8. Fallick C, Sobotka PA, Dunlap ME. Sympathetically mediated changes in capacitance: redistribution of the venous reservoir as a cause of decompensation. Circ Heart Fail. 2011;4(5):669–75.
9. Schrier RW, Abraham WT. Hormones and hemodynamics in heart failure. N Engl J Med. 1999;341(8):577–85.
10. Nohria A, Hasselblad V, Stebbins A, et al. Cardiorenal interactions: insights from the ESCAPE trial. J Am Coll Cardiol. 2008;51(13):1268–74.
11. Ahmed M, Hill J. A rational approach to assess volume status in patients with decompensated heart failure. Curr Heart Fail Rep. 2012;9(2):139–47.
12. West JB, Mathieu-Costello O. Vulnerability of pulmonary capillaries in heart disease. Circulation. 1995;92(3):622–31.

13. Binanay C, Califf RM, Hasselblad V, et al. Evaluation study of congestive heart failure and pulmonary artery catheterization effectiveness: the ESCAPE trial. JAMA. 2005;294(13):1625–33.
14. Thibodeau JT, Turer AT, Gualano SK, et al. Characterization of a novel symptom of advanced heart failure: bendopnea. JACC Heart Fail. 2014;2(1):24–31.
15. Szidon JP. Pathophysiology of the congested lung. Cardiol Clin. 1989;7(1):39–48.
16. Drazner MH, Hamilton MA, Fonarow G, Creaser J, Flavell C, Stevenson LW. Relationship between right and left-sided filling pressures in 1000 patients with advanced heart failure. J Heart Lung Transplant. 1999;18(11):1126–32.
17. Drazner MH, Brown RN, Kaiser PA, et al. Relationship of right- and left-sided filling pressures in patients with advanced heart failure: a 14-year multi-institutional analysis. J Heart Lung Transplant. 2012;31(1):67–72.
18. Nohria A, Tsang SW, Fang JC, et al. Clinical assessment identifies hemodynamic profiles that predict outcomes in patients admitted with heart failure. J Am Coll Cardiol. 2003;41(10):1797–804.
19. Stevenson LW. Are hemodynamic goals viable in tailoring heart failure therapy? Hemodynamic goals are relevant. Circulation. 2006;113(7):1020–7; discussion 1033.
20. Allen LA, Rogers JG, Warnica JW, et al. High mortality without ESCAPE: the registry of heart failure patients receiving pulmonary artery catheters without randomization. J Card Fail. 2008;14(8):661–9.
21. Yancy CW, Jessup M, Bozkurt B, et al. 2013 ACCF/AHA guideline for the management of heart failure: executive summary: a report of the American College of Cardiology Foundation/ American Heart Association Task Force on practice guidelines. Circulation. 2013;128(16):1810–52.
22. Daniels LB, Maisel AS. Natriuretic peptides. J Am Coll Cardiol. 2007;50(25):2357–68.
23. Maisel AS, Krishnaswamy P, Nowak RM, et al. Rapid measurement of B-type natriuretic peptide in the emergency diagnosis of heart failure. N Engl J Med. 2002;347(3):161–7.
24. Januzzi Jr JL, Camargo CA, Anwaruddin S, et al. The N-terminal Pro-BNP investigation of dyspnea in the emergency department (PRIDE) study. Am J Cardiol. 2005;95(8):948–54.
25. Liquori ME, Christenson RH, Collinson PO, Defilippi CR. Cardiac biomarkers in heart failure. Clin Biochem. 2014;47:327–37.
26. Maeda K, Tsutamoto T, Wada A, Hisanaga T, Kinoshita M. Plasma brain natriuretic peptide as a biochemical marker of high

left ventricular end-diastolic pressure in patients with symptomatic left ventricular dysfunction. Am Heart J. 1998;135(5 Pt 1): 825–32.

27. Kazanegra R, Cheng V, Garcia A, et al. A rapid test for B-type natriuretic peptide correlates with falling wedge pressures in patients treated for decompensated heart failure: a pilot study. J Card Fail. 2001;7(1):21–9.

28. Di Angelantonio E, Chowdhury R, Sarwar N, et al. B-type natriuretic peptides and cardiovascular risk: systematic review and meta-analysis of 40 prospective studies. Circulation. 2009; 120(22):2177–87.

29. van Veldhuisen DJ, Linssen GC, Jaarsma T, et al. B-type natriuretic peptide and prognosis in heart failure patients with preserved and reduced ejection fraction. J Am Coll Cardiol. 2013;61(14):1498–506.

30. Redfield MM, Rodeheffer RJ, Jacobsen SJ, Mahoney DW, Bailey KR, Burnett Jr JC. Plasma brain natriuretic peptide concentration: impact of age and gender. J Am Coll Cardiol. 2002;40(5):976–82.

31. Wang TJ, Larson MG, Levy D, et al. Impact of age and sex on plasma natriuretic peptide levels in healthy adults. Am J Cardiol. 2002;90(3):254–8.

32. Wang TJ, Larson MG, Levy D, et al. Impact of obesity on plasma natriuretic peptide levels. Circulation. 2004;109(5):594–600.

33. Drazner MH, de Lemos JA. Unexpected BNP levels in patients with advanced heart failure: a tale of caution and promise. Am Heart J. 2005;149(2):187–9.

34. de Lemos JA, McGuire DK, Drazner MH. B-type natriuretic peptide in cardiovascular disease. Lancet. 2003;362(9380):316–22.

35. O'Neill JO, Bott-Silverman CE, McRae 3rd AT, et al. B-type natriuretic peptide levels are not a surrogate marker for invasive hemodynamics during management of patients with severe heart failure. Am Heart J. 2005;149(2):363–9.

36. Andreassi MG, Del Ry S, Palmieri C, Clerico A, Biagini A, Giannessi D. Up-regulation of 'clearance' receptors in patients with chronic heart failure: a possible explanation for the resistance to biological effects of cardiac natriuretic hormones. Eur J Heart Fail. 2001;3(4):407–14.

37. Goetz KL. Physiology and pathophysiology of atrial peptides. Am J Physiol. 1988;254(1 Pt 1):E1–15.

38. Cuneo RC, Espiner EA, Nicholls MG, Yandle TG, Livesey JH. Effect of physiological levels of atrial natriuretic peptide on hormone secretion: inhibition of angiotensin-induced aldoste-

rone secretion and renin release in normal man. J Clin Endocrinol Metab. 1987;65(4):765–72.

39. Solomon SDB, Bernard E, editors. Essential echocardiography: a practical handbook. Totowa: Humana Press; 2007.

40. Wang L, Lahtinen S, Lentz L, et al. Feasibility of using an implantable system to measure thoracic congestion in an ambulatory chronic heart failure canine model. Pacing Clin Electrophysiol. 2005;28(5):404–11.

41. Abraham WT. Intrathoracic impedance monitoring for early detection of impending heart failure decompensation. Congest Heart Fail (Greenwich, Conn). 2007;13(2):113–5.

42. Yu CM, Wang L, Chau E, et al. Intrathoracic impedance monitoring in patients with heart failure: correlation with fluid status and feasibility of early warning preceding hospitalization. Circulation. 2005;112(6):841–8.

43. Abraham WT, Compton S, Haas G, et al. Intrathoracic impedance vs daily weight monitoring for predicting worsening heart failure events: results of the Fluid Accumulation Status Trial (FAST). Congest Heart Fail (Greenwich, Conn). 2011;17(2):51–5.

44. Small RS, Wickemeyer W, Germany R, et al. Changes in intrathoracic impedance are associated with subsequent risk of hospitalizations for acute decompensated heart failure: clinical utility of implanted device monitoring without a patient alert. J Card Fail. 2009;15(6):475–81.

45. Whellan DJ, Ousdigian KT, Al-Khatib SM, et al. Combined heart failure device diagnostics identify patients at higher risk of subsequent heart failure hospitalizations: results from PARTNERS HF (Program to Access and Review Trending Information and Evaluate Correlation to Symptoms in Patients with Heart Failure) study. J Am Coll Cardiol. 2010;55(17):1803–10.

46. Small RS, Whellan DJ, Boyle A, et al. Implantable device diagnostics on day of discharge identify heart failure patients at increased risk for early readmission for heart failure. Eur J Heart Fail. 2014;16(4):419–25.

47. Whellan DJ, Sarkar S, Koehler J, et al. Development of a method to risk stratify patients with heart failure for 30-day readmission using implantable device diagnostics. Am J Cardiol. 2013;111(1): 79–84.

48. Tang WH, Warman EN, Johnson JW, Small RS, Heywood JT. Threshold crossing of device-based intrathoracic impedance trends identifies relatively increased mortality risk. Eur Heart J. 2012;33(17):2189–96.

49. van Veldhuisen DJ, Braunschweig F, Conraads V, et al. Intrathoracic impedance monitoring, audible patient alerts, and outcome in patients with heart failure. Circulation. 2011;124(16):1719–26.

50. Adamson PB, Magalski A, Braunschweig F, et al. Ongoing right ventricular hemodynamics in heart failure: clinical value of measurements derived from an implantable monitoring system. J Am Coll Cardiol. 2003;41(4):565–71.

51. Magalski A, Adamson P, Gadler F, et al. Continuous ambulatory right heart pressure measurements with an implantable hemodynamic monitor: a multicenter, 12-month follow-up study of patients with chronic heart failure. J Card Fail. 2002;8(2):63–70.

52. Bourge RC, Abraham WT, Adamson PB, et al. Randomized controlled trial of an implantable continuous hemodynamic monitor in patients with advanced heart failure: the COMPASS-HF study. J Am Coll Cardiol. 2008;51(11):1073–9.

53. Ducharme A, Doyon O, White M, Rouleau JL, Brophy JM. Impact of care at a multidisciplinary congestive heart failure clinic: a randomized trial. CMAJ. 2005;173(1):40–5.

54. McAlister FA, Stewart S, Ferrua S, McMurray JJ. Multidisciplinary strategies for the management of heart failure patients at high risk for admission: a systematic review of randomized trials. J Am Coll Cardiol. 2004;44(4):810–9.

55. Walton AS, Krum H. The heartpod implantable heart failure therapy system. Heart Lung Circ. 2005;14 Suppl 2:S31–3.

56. Ritzema J, Melton IC, Richards AM, et al. Direct left atrial pressure monitoring in ambulatory heart failure patients: initial experience with a new permanent implantable device. Circulation. 2007;116(25):2952–9.

57. Ritzema J, Troughton R, Melton I, et al. Physician-directed patient self-management of left atrial pressure in advanced chronic heart failure. Circulation. 2010;121(9):1086–95.

58. Verdejo HE, Castro PF, Concepcion R, et al. Comparison of a radiofrequency-based wireless pressure sensor to swan-ganz catheter and echocardiography for ambulatory assessment of pulmonary artery pressure in heart failure. J Am Coll Cardiol. 2007;50(25):2375–82.

59. Adamson PB, Abraham WT, Aaron M, et al. CHAMPION trial rationale and design: the long-term safety and clinical efficacy of a wireless pulmonary artery pressure monitoring system. J Card Fail. 2011;17(1):3–10.

60. Abraham WT, Adamson PB, Bourge RC, et al. Wireless pulmonary artery haemodynamic monitoring in chronic heart failure: a randomised controlled trial. Lancet. 2011;377(9766):658–66.

61. Ernst ME, Moser M. Use of diuretics in patients with hypertension. N Engl J Med. 2009;361(22):2153–64.
62. Rose BD. Diuretics. Kidney Int. 1991;39(2):336–52.
63. Wargo KA, Banta WM. A comprehensive review of the loop diuretics: should furosemide be first line? Ann Pharmacother. 2009;43(11):1836–47.
64. Ramsay F, Crawford RJ, Allman S, Bailey R, Martin A. An open comparative study of two diuretic combinations, frusemide/amiloride ('Frumil') and bumetanide/potassium chloride ('Burinex' K), in the treatment of congestive cardiac failure in hospital out-patients. Curr Med Res Opin. 1988;10(10):682–9.
65. Felker GM, Lee KL, Bull DA, et al. Diuretic strategies in patients with acute decompensated heart failure. N Engl J Med. 2011;364(9):797–805.
66. Felker GM, Mentz RJ. Diuretics and ultrafiltration in acute decompensated heart failure. J Am Coll Cardiol. 2012;59(24):2145–53.
67. Jentzer JC, DeWald TA, Hernandez AF. Combination of loop diuretics with thiazide-type diuretics in heart failure. J Am Coll Cardiol. 2010;56(19):1527–34.
68. Cohn JN. The management of chronic heart failure. N Engl J Med. 1996;335(7):490–8.
69. Duke M. Thiazide-induced hypokalemia. Association with acute myocardial infarction and ventricular fibrillation. JAMA. 1978;239(1):43–5.
70. Goyal A, Spertus JA, Gosch K, et al. Serum potassium levels and mortality in acute myocardial infarction. JAMA. 2012;307(2):157–64.
71. Pitt B, Zannad F, Remme WJ, et al. The effect of spironolactone on morbidity and mortality in patients with severe heart failure. Randomized Aldactone Evaluation Study Investigators. N Engl J Med. 1999;341(10):709–17.
72. Pitt B, Remme W, Zannad F, et al. Eplerenone, a selective aldosterone blocker, in patients with left ventricular dysfunction after myocardial infarction. N Engl J Med. 2003;348(14):1309–21.
73. Zannad F, McMurray JJ, Krum H, et al. Eplerenone in patients with systolic heart failure and mild symptoms. N Engl J Med. 2011;364(1):11–21.
74. Rossignol P, Menard J, Fay R, Gustafsson F, Pitt B, Zannad F. Eplerenone survival benefits in heart failure patients post-myocardial infarction are independent from its diuretic and potassium-sparing effects. Insights from an EPHESUS (Eplerenone Post-Acute Myocardial Infarction Heart Failure

Efficacy and Survival Study) substudy. J Am Coll Cardiol. 2011;58(19):1958–66.

75. Domanski M, Norman J, Pitt B, Haigney M, Hanlon S, Peyster E. Diuretic use, progressive heart failure, and death in patients in the Studies Of Left Ventricular Dysfunction (SOLVD). J Am Coll Cardiol. 2003;42(4):705–8.

76. Domanski M, Tian X, Haigney M, Pitt B. Diuretic use, progressive heart failure, and death in patients in the DIG study. J Card Fail. 2006;12(5):327–32.

77. Felker GM. Diuretic management in heart failure. Congest Heart Fail (Greenwich, Conn). 2010;16 Suppl 1:S68–72.

78. Hasselblad V, Gattis Stough W, Shah MR, et al. Relation between dose of loop diuretics and outcomes in a heart failure population: results of the ESCAPE trial. Eur J Heart Fail. 2007;9(10):1064–9.

79. Greenberg A, Verbalis JG. Vasopressin receptor antagonists. Kidney Int. 2006;69(12):2124–30.

80. Goldsmith SR, Gheorghiade M. Vasopressin antagonism in heart failure. J Am Coll Cardiol. 2005;46(10):1785–91.

81. Gheorghiade M, Niazi I, Ouyang J, et al. Vasopressin V2-receptor blockade with tolvaptan in patients with chronic heart failure: results from a double-blind, randomized trial. Circulation. 2003;107(21):2690–6.

82. Gheorghiade M, Konstam MA, Burnett Jr JC, et al. Short-term clinical effects of tolvaptan, an oral vasopressin antagonist, in patients hospitalized for heart failure: the EVEREST Clinical Status Trials. JAMA. 2007;297(12):1332–43.

83. Konstam MA, Gheorghiade M, Burnett Jr JC, et al. Effects of oral tolvaptan in patients hospitalized for worsening heart failure: the EVEREST Outcome Trial. JAMA. 2007;297(12):1319–31.

84. Jaski BE, Ha J, Denys BG, Lamba S, Trupp RJ, Abraham WT. Peripherally inserted veno-venous ultrafiltration for rapid treatment of volume overloaded patients. J Card Fail. 2003;9(3):227–31.

85. Costanzo MR, Saltzberg MT, Jessup M, Teerlink JR, Sobotka PA. Ultrafiltration is associated with fewer rehospitalizations than continuous diuretic infusion in patients with decompensated heart failure: results from UNLOAD. J Card Fail. 2010;16(4):277–84.

86. Marenzi G, Lauri G, Grazi M, Assanelli E, Campodonico J, Agostoni P. Circulatory response to fluid overload removal by extracorporeal ultrafiltration in refractory congestive heart failure. J Am Coll Cardiol. 2001;38(4):963–8.

87. Costanzo MR, Guglin ME, Saltzberg MT, et al. Ultrafiltration versus intravenous diuretics for patients hospitalized for acute decompensated heart failure. J Am Coll Cardiol. 2007;49(6): 675–83.
88. Bart BA, Goldsmith SR, Lee KL, et al. Ultrafiltration in decompensated heart failure with cardiorenal syndrome. N Engl J Med. 2012;367(24):2296–304.
89. Mentz RJ, Kjeldsen K, Rossi GP, et al. Decongestion in acute heart failure. Eur J Heart Fail. 2014;16(5):471–82.
90. Sica D. Newer antihypertensive agents. Atlas of Hypertension. Ed. N. Hollenberg. New York: Springer, 2003. p. 301–24.

Index

H.O. Ventura (ed.), *Pharmacologic Trends of Heart Failure*,
Current Cardiovascular Therapy,
DOI 10.1007/978-3-319-30593-6,
© Springer International Publishing Switzerland 2016

Printed in the United States
By Bookmasters